GET YOUR ELBOW OFF THE HORN

GET YOUR ELBOW OFF THE HORN

Stories through the Years

Jack R. Gannon

Gallaudet University Press
Washington, DC

Deaf Lives
A Series Edited by Kristen C. Harmon

Gallaudet University Press
Washington, DC 20002
http://gupress.gallaudet.edu

ISBN (paperback) 978-1-944838-65-2
ISBN (ebook) 978-1-944838-66-9

Library of Congress Cataloging-in-Publication Data

Names: Gannon, Jack R., author.
Title: Get your elbow off the horn : stories through the years / Jack R.
  Gannon.
Description: Washington : Gallaudet University Press, 2020. | Includes
  bibliographical references. | Summary: "A collection of short stories
  about Jack Gannon's life and family. Many of the stories also detail and
  recount Jack's experiences as a student, teacher, and coach at schools
  for the deaf"—Provided by publisher.
Identifiers: LCCN 2019050715 (print) | LCCN 2019050716 (ebook) | ISBN
  9781944838652 (paperback) | ISBN 9781944838669 (ebook)
Subjects: LCSH: Gannon, Jack R. | Teachers of the deaf—United
  States—Biography. | Deaf—Means of communication—United States. |
  American Sign Language.
Classification: LCC HV2426.G36 G36 2020 (print) |
  LCC HV2426.G36 (ebook) | DDC 371.91/2092 [B]—dc23
LC record available at https://lccn.loc.gov/2019050715
LC ebook record available at https://lccn.loc.gov/2019050716

∞ This paper meets the requirements of ANSI/NISO Z39.48-1992
(Permanence of Paper).

Cover and interior design by Eric C. Wilder

To Rosalyn Lee Gannon, with gratitude for making everything possible.

There would be no book and no life without you.

CONTENTS

PART TWO. BECOMING TEACHERS AND COACHES

PART THREE. BECOMING PARENTS

PART FOUR. INTERACTION WITH THE HEARING WORLD AS A DEAF PROFESSIONAL

FOREWORD

Christine L. Gannon

Jack R. Gannon, my father, has dedicated his adult life to the Deaf community. He has been an important leader and activist, a prolific author, and has had many more significant roles in helping improve the lives of Deaf people. He has always staunchly advocated for full access to American Sign Language, for the importance of Deaf role models for younger Deaf youth, and for raising awareness in the hearing world of what Deaf individuals are capable of achieving.

To me, his most important role is that of my father—my "Pops." He has been my dad, my teacher, my support, my editor-in-chief, and my first friend. In our parent-child relationship, I wasn't able to call out to my parents, and as a result, got stuck in a tree longer than the other kids on the block or had other similar unique experiences (some shared in this collection). Still, I have always viewed my father being deaf as a blessing. It provided him with opportunities he otherwise would have missed, including being mentored by many influential Deaf leaders and obtaining a college education that was covered by vocational rehabilitation.

This collection of stories captures many of his poignant experiences as a Deaf man, leader, husband, and father. These memories pay tribute to a great mind that has served my father well and allowed him to give so much to his beloved Deaf community. My hope is that these memories of "the way it was" will be preserved and cherished for their positive messages and insights into the life of this extraordinary Deaf man.

* * *

Jeff D. Gannon

My dad has worked on this book my entire life. Now, just a couple of years away from my fiftieth birthday, I am filled with great gratitude and joy to read his last book. On these pages my dad generously opens his life up for his readers. He shares his confusion and hurt when illness leaves him deaf as an eight-year-old boy. Little did that sweet Ozark hillbilly and Mama's boy know that that moment would open the wide world to him. Within ten years, he became the first in his family to go to college, where he thrived. He fell in love and got married. He became a respected leader, mentor, and historian. He wrote books. He curated a national touring exhibition that was displayed at the Smithsonian Institution and eleven other sites. He played a key advisory role for a PBS documentary about Deaf life in America and was interviewed for the film. He has shaken hands with presidents and traveled the world. He has made a difference.

To me, though, he's Dad. And that's who I want to share with you.

We've always been close, in spite of a few bumps along the way—like when I grew my hair long, wore a black leather jacket, and worked hard to be a rebellious teen. In the grand scope of our time together, that was nothing. Even then, we shared a love of work, of sweat and dirt. We both love old pocketknives, fine tools, pickup trucks, wood split for the fireplace, and a good day's labor. I was probably not more than twelve when my dad had me shimmy twenty-five feet up a large wild cherry tree. I set the rope that controlled the direction the tree would fall when, moments later, my dad took a chainsaw to its base, and I tugged the rope out in the yard.

We lived in Silver Spring, Maryland, the heart of suburbia. But my Dad's hillbilly soul slipped out around the edges—the large garden plot in the backyard, the shed cluttered with planting pots and wood scraps, the woodshop in the basement, the pickup truck in the backyard loaded with mulch. That hillbilly soul, full of grit and determination, runs deep. My Missouri grandfather left school in the third grade after his dad died and started working to help support the family. That hardscrabble man grew up, made a living, and married my grandmother. Together they had four kids, the third being my dad. In 1938 he and his wife packed up their kids and drove to California to work for the war effort. There, my grandmother became one of the original Rosie the Riveters while still managing to care for her four kids. The Gannons have always been tenacious.

Hillbillies make great storytellers, and my dad is no exception. My dad, still a young boy, was a student at the Missouri School for the Deaf (MSD). His family could only afford bus fare at Christmas and summer break, so he mostly lived at school. But those long bus rides were memorable. Young Jack surveyed the other passengers for the most interesting and successful person, maybe a doctor, or a lawyer, he could converse with. He would pull out his notepad and pencil and write, "Hi, my name is Jack. I am deaf. What is your name?" On one of these trips, he was disappointed to learn that his distinguished seatmate was an artist, but he managed to hide his disappointment and continued his conversation. The man was L. L. Broadfoot, a Missouri artist whose work chronicled life in the Ozarks. That day he kindly offered his young friend Jack, along with Jack's classmates, a tour of his studio followed by sandwiches during one of the bus pitstops.

Thus began a lifelong friendship. My dad has always been curious and friendly. He learned from his old friend L. L. Broadfoot that people will always surprise you.

My hillbilly grandfather came up tough. That meant never showing his tender heart, never telling his son how much he loved him. Lucky for Jack Gannon that he met and married Rosalyn Lee. The Lees were an affectionate lot, full of love and hugs for their new son-in-law. Lucky for me, too, because my dad vowed that he would always tell his future children, "I love you," and he would show them too. Lucky for us all, I have never in my life doubted that full heart, that love.

PREFACE

This book is a collection of stories from a lifetime; none of it lived alone. I had the great benefit of caring parents who gave all they had. I had thoughtful teachers, many of whom were Deaf, who encouraged and challenged me. Deaf mentors guided me and gave me the tools to advocate for myself. Chance encounters enlightened me in ways both positive and negative, but the awakening is part of my understanding of human relations. Dear friends have helped in ways more numerous than I can list, especially as I start to slow down. Most of all a loving family has sustained me.

Coming from West Plains, Missouri, a small town in the Ozarks, gave me a sense of identity that stuck with me through all the years. Despite a career that took me many places, I remain tied to the people of those Ozark mountains.

Deep thanks go to the reviewers of the manuscript. Colleagues, friends, and critics, they helped me to better convey stories. Laura Jean Gilbert, Connie Garcia-Barro, and Jean Lindquist Bergey gave feedback on all stories in this collection. In addition, Bobbie Galuska, Mervin D. Garretson, Natalie Gawdiak, Astrid Goodstein, Rae Johnson, Maria Limperic, Molly Luby, Bette Martin, Maureen Nichols, Pete Ripley, Virginia "Ginny" Thompson, and Kathryn Walker offered comments on several of the stories. Their input and critique and occasional nudges to get going pushed this book along. Deaf reviewers could often relate to the experiences described while hearing reviewers gave me a sense of how the text might be interpreted by those just learning about the cultural and linguistic community of Deaf people. Helena Schmitt came to my rescue with technical solutions as computers and programs progressed faster than my ability to keep up. One and all helped the book get to press, and I am deeply grateful for their assistance. That said, I take responsibility for the stories as shared.

Deaf poets added to this book, finding words and patterns that artistically echo the sentiment of the stories. Permission to use the poems came from the poets themselves or their family members if they had passed on. To them, sincere appreciation for the generous sharing.

Ivey Wallace at Gallaudet University Press has given more support than most publishers ever would, simply by remaining interested and supportive of the book. Her friendship has meant a lot over the years.

Jean L. Bergey wrote the introductions to each chapter as well as the about the author statement. Her steady support and friendship has meant a lot and helped get this book to the press.

My most heartfelt gratitude goes to my family. Rosalyn, my wife of sixty years, is the truest of companions on life's journey. She reminded me the book has meaning beyond our family and that it must get done. Rosalyn is the rock of our home, and she has the key to my heart. Our children Jeff and Christine helped with this book in numerous ways, including reviewing stories and offering feedback.

Most importantly, these stories are not mine alone. They are also Rosalyn's, Jeff's, and Christine's. To them go all my love.

PART ONE

BECOMING DEAF AND GOING
AWAY TO SCHOOL

They Say I'm Deaf

They say I'm deaf,
   These folks who call me friend.
   They do not comprehend.

They say I'm deaf,
   And look on me as queer,
Because I cannot hear.

They say I'm deaf,
I, who hear all day
   My throbbing heart at play,
The song the sunset sings,
The joy of pretty things,
   The smiles that greet my eye,
Two lovers passing by,
A brook, a tree, a bird;
Who says I have not heard?
Aye, tho' it must seem odd,
At night I oft hear God.
So many kinds, I get,
   Of happy songs, and yet
   They say I'm deaf!

      —Saul N. Kessler

L ittle is known about Saul N. Kessler (1896–1967), who was believed to be hard of hearing. He was a cartoonist and a poet, and some of his writings appeared in the *Volta Review,* an oral publication, and the *Deaf-Mutes Journal.* This poem appeared in *The Silent Muse, An Anthology of Prose and Poetry by the Deaf* published by the Gallaudet College Alumni Association in 1960.

INTRODUCTION

Born at home on November 23, 1936, not far from West Plains, Missouri, Jack Randle Gannon grew up in a rural setting with his parents and three siblings. His father worked as an automobile mechanic, his mother as a homemaker who also worked in a shoe store on the town square in West Plains. The family's home used water from a well that was almost a football field away from the house, and it was one of Jack's chores to draw the water and carry the buckets. He credits this assignment with giving him the strength to beat his first-year Gallaudet classmates at arm wrestling, thus gaining some athletic credibility with older students.

Jack was seven years old in 1943 when his parents moved the family to Richmond, California, to gain wartime factory jobs. A year later, in 1944, Jack became deaf from spinal meningitis. His parents moved him from one oral program to another, never satisfied with the results. It was not until Jack's father met a custodian from the California School for the Deaf (CSD) in Berkeley that the family considered sending him to a school for deaf students. Jack went, but only for a few months. By 1945 World

War II had ended, and along with it, so did job opportunities. The family returned to their Ozark home.

A CSD teacher recommended the Missouri School for the Deaf (MSD) for Jack. From 1946 until 1954, he attended the school in Fulton, Missouri, staying there for weeks at a time, returning home only for winter and summer breaks. At MSD, Jack came to know and appreciate the community of Deaf people surrounding the school, particularly the Deaf teachers.

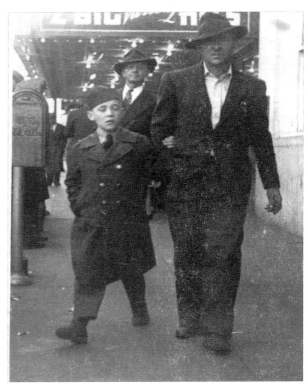

My father and me.

5

MY BRIEF JOURNEY THROUGH
THE HEARING WORLD

Rain tinkled gently on our tin roof, one of my favorite sounds. On a rainy day, I often would get a sheet and, with my mother's help, put it over the dining room table. I would crawl under the makeshift tent and lay there on the floor, listening to what I considered music, the most beautiful sound in my fleeting hearing world.

The woods surrounding our home abounded with sounds. The trees attracted a wide variety of birds with their calls, quarrels, and songs. At night frogs croaked in the nearby pond. Crickets chirped, katydids rubbed their wings together, and insects buzzed against the metal screens trying to get to the light inside the house. In the evenings, the family often gathered around the radio to keep up with the news from the rest of the world. Dad's favorite gadget played 1940s tunes and radio shows such as *Terry and the Pirates,* and other programs.

Listening to the tinkle of the rain, these were all the most beautiful but fleeting sounds in my brief journey through the hearing world. I wondered what I would be like when I grew up. What was I meant to be?

I was soon to find out.

My mother, father, sister Betty Jo, brother Frank Lester, and me (age one).

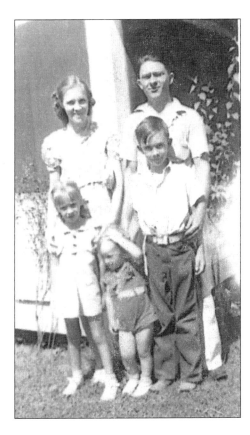

HOW DO YOU MAKE HANDS TALK?

I must have been about six years old the day Frank Lester, my older brother, came home with the news that he had seen some deaf people downtown on "The Square," talking with their hands.

Our mouths dropped open. "What?!" we exclaimed in unison. The Square was the business district of West Plains, our small southern Missouri hometown. In the center of The Square stood a huge, four-story white stone courthouse with black screened windows on the top floor. Everyone knew that these windows were where the county jail was because mothers would point upward in that direction and tell their small children, "If you don't behave, they will put you *up there*!"

The main thoroughfare through town circled The Square from which roads jutted out in four directions—north, east, south, and west. Around the circle was where the town's main business district was located—hence The Square's name.

Saturdays and Mondays were the busiest days of the week on The Square. On Mondays, the local farmers brought their livestock to the market. On Saturdays, it seemed, everyone flocked to town to do their shopping, pay their bills, attend the "picture show," or just sit around The Square and visit.

It was on a Saturday that my brother Frank Lester encountered those deaf people talking with their hands on The Square. Curious, we listened attentively as he described what he saw. He had been part of a small crowd that had stopped to gawk at the deaf persons. He said he could not understand one word they had said, but it was obvious that they understood each other because of the way they nodded their heads in response and laughed. And, he said, they seemed to talk so fast.

As a boxer.

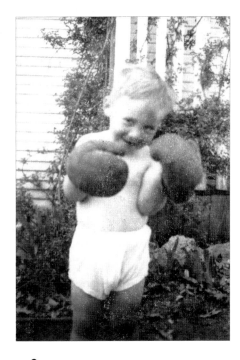

That was my introduction to deaf people. Until that day, I hadn't known there were deaf people in the world. I was fascinated. Imagine *talking with your hands*! I sat there at the table and looked down at my hands and studied them intently.

"How do you make hands talk?" I asked the family. "Where's the mouth?"

"There's no mouth, stupid!" my brother said, throwing up his hands before he tried to describe how the deaf people had talked: by gesturing wildly. They stood in a circle watching each other, he explained. One would use his hands and arms to "talk" while the others watched. My brother said that they moved their fingers very rapidly, too, and it looked as if they were writing a message in the air, and then they would move their hands and arms about their body with very expressive faces. Frank Lester waved his arms about his body in different directions, imitating what he had seen. And, he said again, that as he watched, he could see that they understood each other by their facial expressions and the way they nodded their heads. He said they signed so fast he had no idea how a person could see and understand everything that was being signed.

"Gosh," I said, amazed. "I sure wish I could do that!" I hadn't the slightest idea how soon that wish would come true.

INTO A NEW SOUNDLESS WORLD

During World War II, my parents accepted good-paying jobs at the shipyards in California to contribute to America's war effort. We put our house and property, Ten Rocky Acres, up for rent, and our family of five made the trek across the country in our 1936 Chevrolet with what possessions we could take. We secured housing in a large housing development constructed for shipyard employees in Richmond, California. It was there that I became gravely ill.

Those were the years before the polio vaccination had been discovered, and my mother feared I had contracted polio. I developed a raging fever, but, for some reason, was not allowed any liquids. My Aunt Babe would bring me a wet washcloth to put on my forehead, and when no one was looking, I would suck what moisture I could from the washcloth in an attempt to quench my terrible thirst. When I did not get any better, Mom and Dad took me to a hospital far from home. My illness was diagnosed eventually as spinal meningitis. During an operation at the hospital, the doctors and nurses bent me over into a ball and inserted long medical needles into my back. I never pinpointed exactly when my hearing disappeared. I was eight years old.

One day, about a week after I returned home from the hospital, the local ice cream vendor drove by, and along with the other neighborhood kids, I ran to get an ice cream bar. As I handed over money for the ice cream, the vendor spoke to me, and I thought it strange that I could not understand what he said. When I went back home, I told Mom what had happened. "Mom," I said, "The ice cream man talked to me, and I didn't understand what the man said to me."

"I told you, Jack," Mom said resignedly, a hurt look on her face. "I told you, you are deaf!"

I nodded my head and said, "Oh," and wandered off. I did not fully understand what she was talking about, or what she meant, but I have always remembered that incident because that was the beginning of my conscious journey into the world of silence.

Gradually I came to realize that my illness had thrust me into a strange, new world, a world I did not understand nor want to be part of. That journey helped me understand what being deaf really is, what it meant to an individual, and how it impacted our lives. I would learn the answers gradually over a lifetime. And, I would learn, like so many others before me, not only how to "survive" in a world of sound, but how to appreciate and reap the benefits of both worlds.

Being deaf means many things for me. First of all, being profoundly deaf means almost total exclusion from the world of sound . . . that world of music; free-flowing, spoken conversation; background noises and distant sounds. It means living in two worlds: the world of sound and the world of silence. Being deaf means teaching your eyes to "listen" and your hands to talk. It means learning to speak words and sounds you cannot hear. As a newly deaf person, I was always relying on my vision to "hear," to receive, to understand, and to be aware of what was being said or happening. No longer could I do one thing and be consciously aware of something else going on unless it was within my scope of vision. At times, being deaf can mean loneliness, isolation even in a crowd. It meant, for me, turning inward and thriving on my own thoughts, fantasies, and dreams. It meant falling in love with books and learning to keep myself entertained. When we returned to Ten Rocky Acres, our home, no more would I hear the slamming of our neighbor's screen door, the moaning and screeching sound of a rusty sign in the wind near the highway over the hill, the gentle tinkle of the rain on the tin roof, the chirps of the cicadas and crickets, the croaks of the frogs down by the pond, the insects' buzzing as they popped against the window screens, the sighing of trees as the wind ruffled their leaves and they bowed in the breeze. The radio that had been our link to the world and the center of the family attention had, for me, become just a wooden box.

Becoming deaf for me meant a loss of fluent, easy, comfortable verbal communication. It meant struggling with the spoken word, trying to understand words on unmoving lips and studying, searching facial expressions, body movements, and gestures for clues that might help put the verbal puzzle together. It meant struggling to produce sounds I could no longer hear and write a language that had rules and rules and rules that made little sense. And, for me, it meant being left out, most of the time unintentionally of course, of the family and my friends and group conversations. It meant learning to accept and ignore the rude, quick brush-off when a person learned you were deaf. It meant being labeled and sometimes feeling "abnormal," "different," "broken," "freakish," "idiotic," "dumb," and "deaf-mute"—even though I could still speak.

Most disturbingly, it meant enduring attempts to become "normal." Over and over, I was told that a deaf person *must* not sign and *must* learn to talk and lipread "because it is a hearing world out there!" I had to fit into *their* world with no regard, respect, nor acceptance of *my* world. I was the one who had to be "fixed."

When I was sent to a school for deaf students, my life began to take on meaning, and I began to understand. I learned that there were others like me and that by becoming deaf at eight years of age, I was more fortunate than many because I had heard spoken language before becoming deaf. I learned to talk with my hands and discovered a beautiful, new comfortable world of silent, expressive communication. I found a place where I could belong, be involved, and have the opportunity to thrive and learn and grow into the individual that I am. I had started down the road to understanding and accepting who I was. By the time I

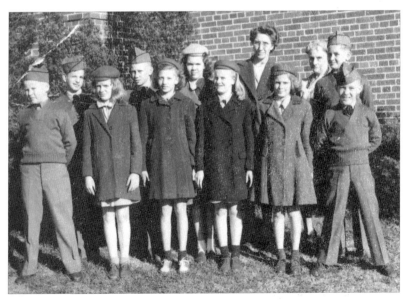

My second-grade class at Stark Hall, MSD, in 1947
(I'm in the front row farthest right).

graduated from school, I had come to realize that I was as normal as anyone else, even if I could no longer hear.

I was in a class where the other students were just like me. I was exposed to teachers trained to work with deaf and hard of hearing children; in fact, many were deaf themselves. I found it easy to relate to these deaf teachers and looked up to many of them. Some became my role models and inspiration. Challenging me, they became the people I would learn to love and admire and who, in many different ways, left a tremendous impact on my life. Most of my deaf teachers became lifelong friends. For the first time since I had become deaf, I felt perfectly normal.

I also came to realize that there was nothing wrong with being deaf; we were just different. Even so, being deaf meant we had to learn to live in a world that relied heavily on sound. The radio, public announcements, news broadcasts, and conversation—all were inaccessible to me.

While school had opened a new world to me, I had to learn with the limitations imposed on me, trying to keep pace with the hearing world by lipreading. My speech was quite understandable, but lipreading was terribly restrictive and frustrating. I caught no more than 25 percent of the words that appeared on the lips. My friends and I always looked forward to going home, but going back to the "hearing environment" also reminded us of our frustration associated with living in a world that was so unnecessarily ignorant about deaf people. I was determined that in some way I would find a way and help change that.

As an adult, being deaf has meant an ongoing struggle with paternalistic, condescending, and ignorant attitudes. I have had to deal with people who looked down on me or viewed me as inferior simply because they could hear, and I could not. I have lived with and been exposed to teachers, educators, and parents who believed that the solution was simply to teach deaf individuals to talk and lipread. This journey is strewn with rocks and boulders of ignorance and paternalistic and "fix-it" attitudes. There is bitterness, heartbreak, and family hostility. But I have had a good life because I have had the good fortune to meet so many dedicated, committed, wonderful, talented people. These individuals have enriched my life. Despite all the negativity, I had the good fortune to find a world of beauty, an appreciative world rich in history, heritage, language, and uniquely our own. It is also a world of silent poetry, humor, stories of human perseverance, and success against the odds. It has been a heartwarming journey.

AUNT EVA AND MY MISSED MIRACLE

Most people who became deaf as children or in their early teens can recount stories of their parents' or relatives' futile search for a miracle to restore their hearing. I read a story about a young girl who was taken aloft in an airplane that went through a steep dive in an effort to "clear her ears" and another about a professional boxer who parachuted out of an airplane. Both stories had unfortunate endings—neither became hearing.

Many of my deaf friends remember being dragged from one doctor or expensive clinic to another in search of that elusive cure. Unlike many of them, however, I was taken to a revivalist. Preachers, I guess, were cheaper. I must have been ten years old the summer a revivalist came to our small southern Missouri town, promising cures. It was one of those Bible-thumping, fist-shaking, people-weeping revivals where the man of God promised to cure everything from a hangnail to people who couldn't walk. I saw a man who had been unable to walk, rise up, hobble forward, and walk back!

Aunt Eva was Cousin Jimmy's mother. Jimmy was one year older than me, and we were best friends. He was a very considerate person who always exhibited much patience when talking with me. Aunt Eva was a thin, petite woman with jet black hair, and was one of the most religious members of our clan. She and her husband, Uncle Roy, had always exhibited a keen interest in my deafness. When the revival came to town, Aunt Eva got my parents' permission to take me. The only problem was—as usual—no one bothered to tell me what was going on. I thought I was just being taken to another boring religious service where I could not understand anything.

Jimmy and his sisters went with me to the church down by the creek, and I noticed Jimmy behaving in an unusual, uncomfortable way. It was a hot, humid July night, and the preacher was quite long-winded. I quickly became bored and started squirming restlessly on the hard, wooden chair. To pass the time, my eyes wandered around. The windows were raised as far as they could go, but no air came through. Summer insects, attracted by the lights, buzzed against the screens. I remembered how noisy it was as their wings kept zapping against the wire barrier that had been made to keep them out. A sea of handheld fans fluttered throughout the room. All the movement was a welcome distraction. Other young children fidgeted restlessly next to their parents. Elderly men chewed tobacco that they spat in cans they had brought with them. Others dozed.

Near the end of the service, I gazed as the first wave of people went forward to meet with the preacher. It was then that I saw the man hobble up and walk back. Others went forward and seemed to feel better when they returned because there were smiles on their faces. Suddenly, Aunt Eva, sitting next to me, stood up, grabbed hold of my arm, and yanked me forward. I was startled by the movement, and the idea of walking before all those staring eyes frightened me. I shook my head no, but Aunt Eva dragged me toward the pulpit. I glanced over my shoulder and saw Jimmy make a quick exit out the door. Apparently, he wanted nothing to do with whatever was going on. I watched as Aunt Eva talked to the preacher, probably telling him what was "wrong" with me.

The preacher looked at me sternly, pointed his finger to the floor, and spoke. I looked at the floor then up at him, trying to figure out what he was saying. He put his hands on my shoulders and pushed downward, shoving me into a kneeling position. It was then that I understood what he wanted me to do. I turned my head and watched Aunt Eva return to her seat. The preacher hooked one hand under my chin and pulled my head up to look into his face, telling me to pay attention. He then placed one hand on top of my head and raised his other hand. I looked up, trying to lipread what he was saying, but he pushed my head back down. For what seemed like an eternity, I knelt there looking at the floor, feeling his hand on top of my head shake and move, wondering all the while what was going on around me. The wooden floor hurt my knees. I was very uncomfortable and wished I were somewhere else. Even sitting on that hard pew watching the insects hit the screen, I realized, was better than this. I was tempted to get up and run out of the church, but the preacher's hand held me firmly in place.

I was to learn later from my cousin that the preacher shouted and begged God to forgive all my sins and restore my hearing. When nothing happened, he placed both of his hands over my ears and began shaking my head in different directions. The movement made me dizzy, and the room started to dance around me. Still, nothing happened. The preacher then put his index fingers in each ear and pushed inward roughly before grasping my ears and yanking them outwards. All this time, he was praying furiously, his eyes shut, and shouting to God to restore my hearing. God and I must have had a special kinship at that moment. Neither of us was listening.

Behind me, the congregation prayed, moaned, and begged. Many had their arms raised, and they shook their clenched fists heavenward. Some people were even on their knees in the aisle.

Others, including Aunt Eva, were crying. "Amen! Amen! Amen!" they shouted in unison, on cue.

But nothing happened.

After what seemed like forever, the preacher finally grabbed my shoulders and pulled me up, and I looked into a very disappointed, sweaty face. He turned me around and gave me a gentle shove in the direction of my chair. I was embarrassed and upset by the experience. I returned to my seat as deaf as I was when I left it.

As my aunt described what had happened as I was in the preacher's hands, she raised her shoulders, the palms of her hands upward, and shook her head dejectedly and said matter of factly, "The preacher said he couldn't cure you because you didn't have enough faith."

How could I have faith, I wondered to myself, when nobody had bothered to tell me what was going on?

AWAY TO SCHOOL

I sat alone hunched on the little chair next to the narrow bed in my new dormitory room and cried.

"Why, Jack! You're crying!" Miss Davis said when she found me, her eyes wide and her brows furrowed. She had put a soft hand on my shoulder to get my attention. And then she crouched in front of me so that her face was directly opposite mine as she crisply mouthed the words. Looking sad, she put an index finger to her eyes and slowly ran them down her cheeks. What she said struck me as dumb—wasn't it obvious that I was crying, and didn't I already know that?! Miss Davis then straightened up, bent her arms, and placed her fists on her hips. She shook her head in a sympathetic yet disapproving manner, and smiled. Her face and body language told me that this is no place for tears.

My parents and younger brother Donnie had just left on the long journey back home . . . without me. I'm sure that my mother had explained all this to me—that they were taking me away to school, but at that early age, the details hadn't registered. I had no idea what I was doing in this new place or what lay ahead for me, and at that moment, I felt abandoned in a strange, new world. I was nine years old.

Back home, a school was one large room in a white clapboard schoolhouse with a large potbellied stove, a playground, two outhouses, and a well with a hand pump for our drinking water. Here at MSD, I was in a huge, new, brick building that had indoor plumbing and restrooms, with rows of gleaming white sinks, shower stalls, and shiny waxed granite floors. Later I would learn the building was named Stark Hall in honor of Governor Lloyd Crow Stark. At that moment, though, I had no idea what I'd done to deserve such punishment, and I didn't want any part of this new world.

Miss Davis was the head houseparent or supervisor, as they were called in those days, at Stark Hall, the school's primary unit for young children. She wore round wire-rimmed glasses, and her hair was braided and rolled into an old-fashioned bun that sat on the back of her head. Although she was slightly taller, in many ways, she resembled my gentle, frail grandmother.

Getting no response from me, Miss Davis sat down on the bed next to me, placed her hand on my knee, and asked, "Why are you crying, Jack?" Her question surprised me. Was I doing something unheard of? In reality, Miss Davis had this routine down pat, for she had gone through it countless times. Every fall, she dealt with heartbroken children who had been wrenched away from their families for the first time.

To Miss Davis, MSD was not a place for sadness. Here children learned, had fun, developed new friendships, and shared a togetherness that, for many, would last a lifetime. It was designed for deaf children who could not communicate in the hearing world around them and often within their own families. Here at MSD, they would meet trained, understanding, knowledgeable teachers and houseparents and start down the path of learning among peers. They would establish their own identity, develop speech and language skills, and learn to communicate, in some cases, for the first time. School opened the minds of young deaf children.

"We're so happy to have you with us, Jack," Miss Davis said, making me feel like someone special. She took a hankie from her bra, and wiped away my tears. "You're just going to love it here! You're going to make many new friends! You're going to have lots of fun!" she assured me as she crossed her hands and put them over her heart, making the sign LOVE. "C'mon now," she said, taking me by the hand and pulling me up from the chair. "I want you to meet some new friends."

As I rose, a tall skinny kid with two long front teeth bounced into the room and spoke to Miss Davis. She held up her hand to tell him to stop talking and introduced us. D-A-L-E, she moved her fingers as she mouthed each letter. Dale thrust his bony hand forward and shook mine. I was surprised because Dale, a second-year student, talked just like me. I eventually learned he was what they called "hard of hearing." Unlike me and most of the other kids who were deaf, Dale could hear fairly well, and I was told, had very good speech. He also knew how to use his hands to talk. Dale and I were placed in the same class and became good friends. He helped me get acquainted with other students. He taught me my first sign. When he pointed to a chair and signed CHAIR, I picked it up right away. I was amazed at how easy it was to learn a sign.

With Miss Davis's encouragement, Dale showed me around Stark Hall. It was a three-story, self-contained unit where the younger children ate, slept, and attended classes. It was designed in a square with a paved play area in the center. One wing housed the girls' residence hall, and the opposite wing housed the boys' rooms, with classrooms and offices in between. The building had a dining room and kitchen, a small auditorium-gymnasium, and indoor play areas in the basement. On the stairwell landing of each floor was a small carved, wooden bear—Missouri's mascot—which I would learn later had been carved by a graduate of the school. I was awed as Dale led me from one area of the building to the next. Its size overwhelmed me.

Each dormitory room had four beds, one in each corner. Next to each bed stood a wooden wardrobe with a door, and inside each wardrobe was a mirror, a shelf for soap and a toothbrush, and a bar for towels. Each wardrobe had a set of drawers and a place to put our shoes and hang our clothes. Overhead was an enclosed compartment for our suitcases.

Pointing to the enclosed overhead compartments, with a scary face and imitating a ghost's ghoulish movements, Don, one of my new roommates, said just before we went to bed that night, "That's where the ghosts are." I had not grown up believing much in ghosts, but coming to a strange new place was an adventure for me, and I was no longer sure of anything.

That first night away from home, after the lights went out, I pulled the bed covers up tightly around my chin and kept a wary, watchful eye on those doors, until I finally drifted off to sleep from exhaustion, tears rolling down my cheeks. I missed my dog Deadeye, my brothers and sister, and Mom and Dad.

MY NAME BECOMES A LABEL

One of the most striking differences between attending a residential school and the local public school was a thing called labels. Each year as "label time" arrived at our house, during the first part of August, Mom would go to the store and buy a special kind of indelible black ink. She then would get a white cloth—usually an old bed sheet—and start writing my name repeatedly on it. Next, she would cut the piece of cloth into small, narrow, rectangular pieces and sew by hand each piece to each item of new clothing she had bought for me.

This tedious ritual occurred throughout my school years, yet Mom never seemed to mind. When I saw Mom get out her sewing basket and the labels, I knew my summer vacation was almost over, and a new academic year stretched out ahead. I had labels on everything: socks, shirts, pants, caps, coat, and underwear. If the Trailways bus that took us to school had taken a wrong turn, wound up in St. Louis, and dropped us off in a crowd, we couldn't have gotten lost—we were too well-labeled!

These labels, of course, prevented our clothes from getting mixed up in the school laundry. On laundry day, one of the older students would drive the old school pickup truck from dormitory to dormitory, collect all the bags of dirty clothes, and transport them to the school laundry facility. After the garments were washed and neatly folded, they would be returned to each dorm where the houseparents separated and distributed them into each student's clothes box.

The labels served other useful purposes, too. They allowed us to meet and become acquainted with newcomers. In the fall, when a new kid arrived, if he or she could not sign or talk or did not know his or her name—and many young deaf kids didn't— the houseparent or one of the older kids would walk up to the new student, grab the kid's shirt collar, fold it back, read his or her name, and then sign and fingerspell to the rest of us: THAT'S s-m-i-t-h. Sometimes the houseparent or an older kid would, at the same time, give the new kid a name sign right there on the spot. That name sign—good or bad—usually stuck like a label for the rest of the student's school life and even into adulthood.

This practice of labeling, no doubt, inspired the following amusing exchange I witnessed as an adult one summer in a hotel lounge at a national convention of deaf people.

Two deaf men met after a long separation. They were former schoolmates who had not seen each other for years. After giving each other the typical bear hug, they stood back and inspected one another. Then, pretending not to remember each other's name, they pointed at each other and signed, NAME YOU WHAT?

FORGOT, signed the first. He went through the routine of thinking, then suddenly, his face brightened, and he held up an index finger indicating he had a bright idea, "Wait!" He reached behind his neck, folded back his shirt collar, turned his head backward in that direction where the school name labels were always attached, and pretended to read it.

NAME MINE S-E-A-R-S, he fingerspelled.

OH, signed the second one, going through the same motions, and after pretending to read his name label, he responded: NAME MINE A-R-R-O-W.

MY SISTER, AN ANGEL

When I arrived home from MSD that first Christmas break, my brother Frank Lester and sister Betty Jo were still in school. Betty persuaded me to attend school with them the next day, and I liked the thought of visiting my former school classmates and friends. So the next day, we trudged that long country mile to Renfro on the Gainsville Route.

The old Renfro schoolhouse, sitting on a hill above the highway curve, was a familiar sight. We passed the hill between the playground and the highway. I smiled to myself as I remembered pushing Frank and his pal, Billy Joe, over the embankment as they grappled in a wrestling match. The water pump stood at the front of the schoolyard, not far from the flagpole. Behind the white clapboard building stood the two outdoor privies, one for boys and one for girls. Next to the back door stood cords and cords of oak that farmers had brought. These logs fed the huge potbelly stove in the front of the room. Inside, the whole school shone with Christmas cheer. There was a strong smell of cedar, and long lines of green and red construction paper chains hung from the walls. Holly and pine needles scented the air. Threaded popcorn circled the fat cedar Christmas tree in the front corner of the room. Next to it was a temporary stage built for the annual Christmas play, and above the tree, a wire ran from wall to wall. Over it, bedsheets and blankets had been pinned to serve as curtains. Because of the weight, the line was propped up with two clothesline poles, one on each side of the stage.

As was typical in those one-room schoolhouses, the children sat in rows by grade, and a single teacher taught all nine grades. I sat at a vacant desk behind my sister, unable to hear or understand anything. I felt self-conscious and nervous, played with a pencil, and watched it roll down the slanted desktop until my sister turned around and put her finger to her lips and whispered, "Shhhh!" I hadn't realized that the rolling pencil made noise. I realized just then how difficult it was to communicate with my peers compared to MSD. They could understand what I said, but lipreading them was hit or miss, and I did not always understand, so I would repeat what I thought they had said to be sure I was following them. They would look at me as a deaf person.

After recess, the teacher gathered the members of the Christmas pageant cast together to practice their lines and gave the rest of the students busy work. I sat there at the desk bored, watching the students practice their lines, not able to follow one word. The teacher noticed my restlessness and came over to talk with me. I lipread her the best I could and repeated the words she spoke to be sure I was following. She told me, pointing to the stage, "Your sister is an angel."

"An angel?" I repeated, not realizing how loud I spoke. I had just become deaf, and I was still very shy and self-conscious. I also had not yet learned to control the volume of my voice. Everyone in the room turned to look at me as soon as I spoke, much to my mortification. Although the teacher tried to console me, I burst into tears.

For years after that embarrassing experience, I kept my voice low when speaking in crowds, with my hearing friends always prodding me, "Speak up, Jack, I can't hear you."

Visiting my family for Christmas (I'm in the military uniform).

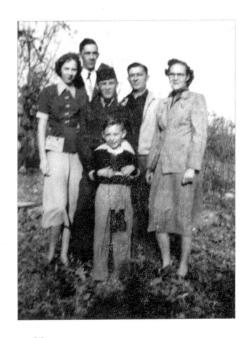

TALK! TALK! TALK!

Heavy emphasis was placed on teaching deaf children speech during my school days. The use of sign language was frowned on or forbidden in most schools during that time. Many hearing educators believed that the use of sign language interfered with the acquisition and development of spoken language, even though research has come to prove the opposite. For that reason and due to the lack of sign language classes, my parents and brothers and sister never learned to sign.

Mrs. McQueen was our teacher from the first through the third grades at Stark Hall. She must have been in her sixties the day I joined the class. She was a tall, willowy, bespectacled woman with slightly stooped shoulders and silver hair. She had long, narrow feet and a pointed nose. A strict disciplinarian, she was also a devoted teacher and a tender, loving, caring person. Inside her thin body, my classmates and I knew, was a heart of pure gold. But what I remember best about Mrs. McQueen's physique was her mouth. A good deal of our class time was devoted to learning speech, and that was how I became so well acquainted with Mrs. McQueen's gold-capped teeth, her dental bridges, fillings, and the shape of her mouth because that was the part of her body I spent the most time looking at . . . and into.

"Talk! Talk! Talk!" was the familiar old refrain we were told over and over again.

During speech class, my classmates and I would put on our big individual earphones and gather in a semicircle. Mrs. McQueen would stand in the center of the semicircle with the speech vowel chart on her left. With a microphone in one hand and a wooden pointer in the other, she would lead us through the speech chart: "A-e-i-o-u . . . a-e-i-o-u . . . a-a-a-a-a . . . e-e-e-e-e . . . i-i-i-i-i . . . o-o-o-o-o . . . u-u-u-u-u . . ." we would go in unison. Watching my classmates go through the vowel chart always reminded me of a cat meowing.

After the group session, Mrs. McQueen would give us our class assignments, and then call each of us forward, one by one, to work on our individual weaknesses. We would sit or stand in front of her with our earphones clamped over our heads and the electrical cord dangling down our bodies to the plug where it was connected to our individual audio boxes. We would listen to the sounds she made and try to imitate them. Since I could hear nothing, the dial on my box was always turned up full blast, and I could feel a buzzing, scratchy sensation in my ears. Whatever sound she made it always came through as "Bzzzzz . . . bzzzzz . . . bzzzzz." Mrs. McQueen would point to the chart, demonstrate how a particular letter sound was made, and then ask me to repeat it. When I did not get the sound right she would place the pointer under her armpit, take one of my hands and place it somewhere on her face where I could best feel the vibrations, and ask me to copy her. We would repeat this process over and over again and again until she was satisfied . . . or gave up.

The "sh" sound was my weakness. "Sh- sh- sh- sh . . ." Mrs. McQueen repeatedly pronounced that sound, holding my hand to her chin as I watched her mouth movement.

"S-h-h-h . . . s-h-h-h . . . s-h-h-h . . ." I tried to imitate her. "No, no, no, Jack," she would respond, "Sh- . . . sh- . . . sh-. . . ." and I would try again. "S-h-h-h . . . s-h-h-h . . . s-h-h-h. . . ." "No, no, no . . . sh- . . . sh- . . . sh. . . ."

Next came the rapid rattle of the k-k-k-k-k sound, easily the leading spittle producer. Mrs. McQueen's tongue would curl up and touch the roof of her mouth in a movement that resembled the arch of a frightened cat's back. She would place my hand under her chin and close to her throat so I could feel her tongue jumping up and down, up and down, up and down. "K-k-k-k-k . . ." Mrs. McQueen went as her tongue repeatedly bounced off the roof of her mouth. "K-k-k-k-k . . ." I copied, wiping the wetness from my face. Next, Mrs. McQueen placed my fingers on the side of her nose to give me the nasal feeling of the letter "n" and pronounced it, "n . . . n . . . n . . . n . . . n . . ." I thought I was pretty good with that one because my oldest brother had told me one day, "Jack, do you realize that you talk through your nose?"

The speech drills were long and tedious, mainly because I could not hear the results of my efforts and had no way of judging my progress. Like the other kids, I soon became bored with the monotonous repetition, and my attention would begin to drift. When I became distracted, as I often did, the teacher would gently nudge me or grasp my chin in her hand and draw my attention back to the speech lesson.

As might be expected, my classmates' speech abilities varied greatly. Those who became deaf after hearing sound generally had better speech than those who were born deaf and had never heard any sound or became deaf before they developed a language. Some of the students used their speech skills with family and close friends. Some used them in public. Many—including graduates of the prominent oral schools—never used their speech skills after they left school once they realized, after repeated attempts, how unreliable it was. It's no wonder sign language has been so popular with so many deaf people.

"LONG TOOTH," "PULL-UP-PANTS," AND OTHER NAME SIGNS

Most deaf people I have known who use sign language have name signs. A name sign, as the words imply, is a sign or signs for a person's name. It is a hand movement that establishes the person's identity and eliminates the need to fingerspell a name over and over again. Name signs are very helpful when attempting to catch a deaf person's attention across the table or in another part of the room, and they are especially useful if a person has a long, hard-to-spell last name like "Horjeovnzk." Most individuals with short names like "Lee" or "Hall" do not have or need a name sign because those names are so easy to fingerspell.

Most name signs are created and bestowed by an older deaf person, usually the offspring of deaf parents. Sometimes a houseparent or a teacher may give a new student a name sign, but whether it sticks depends on the student's peers and whether they use it. It is considered both a tradition and an honor to be given a name sign, and it is not considered culturally acceptable for a newcomer—especially a hearing person—to demand or create their own name sign.

Some name signs are made with letters of the manual alphabet. For example, "BB" was the initialized name sign of the late Bernard Bragg, the internationally known deaf actor and one of the founders of the National Theatre of the Deaf. "BBB" (note the number of Bs) was the name sign of the late Byron B. Burnes, a distinguished national leader who served as president of the National Association of the Deaf and for whom a building on the Gallaudet University Northwest campus was named. "JJ" was the initialized name sign of Jerald M. Jordan, the first deaf American to become president of the Committee International des Sports des Sourds (International Committee of Sports for the Deaf). "TJ" (using both the letters "T" and "J" simultaneously) was the identity of Terrence J. O'Rourke, a successful author and book publisher.

Some deaf individuals may have two or three or even four name signs during their lifetime. Their name sign may change as they grow older and may change again when they leave school. At a leadership training program in Switzerland, I met two young women who still used their childhood name signs BROWN CURL and RED CURL. A few deaf people may choose to create or modify their own name signs for various reasons, much like hearing people modify their nicknames or names (from "Bobby" to "Robert," for example).

In some deaf families, a name sign is handed down from one generation to the next, and some use the same body placement for a name sign while using a different letter for each member of the family, giving it a family homogeneity. An example of this could be "D-on-the-chest" for Don, the father, "C-on-the-chest" for Cora, the mother, and "F-on-the-chest" for their daughter, Frannie. Some parents and their offspring have the same sign with "little" or "big" added to differentiate between the child and the adult, "Little F" for Frank Jr. and "Big F" for Frank Sr. for example.

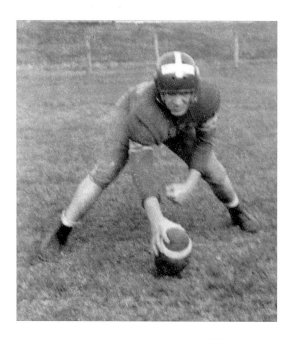

As a football center with "Don't Tread on Me" on my helmet!

Some name signs illustrate a physical feature (which, incidentally, is not always complimentary) or a characteristic behavioral trait, or a play on the name, or its sound, or how it is spelled. In college, we had an English professor named Dr. Siger. His name sign? "Cigar," of course, because of the sound resemblance. Another professor's name was Mr. Scouten. His name sign was the Boy Scout sign and salute. A female student whose last name happened to be Lefkow took a lot of teasing from her college mates who gave her the name sign of "Left Cow." Yerker Andersson, former president of the World Federation of the Deaf, had the name sign of "pipe" (the manual alphabet letter "Y" placed in the corner of the mouth imitating a pipe) because for a long time he smoked a pipe. He gave up smoking, but his pipe name sign endures.

At Gallaudet University, most name signs were dropped, and last names were fingerspelled because there were too many identical name signs. Only a few—mostly leaders—continued to be recognized by their personal name signs.

When I arrived at MSD, I was given the name sign of "G" moving down from the forehead to the chin. I think Miss Davis, my houseparent, gave it to me, and I have had the same name sign all my life. It is a name sign I am proud to share with Dr. W. Ted Griffing and Gary Malkowski. Dr. Griffing was for many years a popular teacher at the Oklahoma School for the Deaf, the editor of *The Deaf Oklahoman,* and a wonderful, folksy writer. Gary

Malkowski made news when he became the first deaf person ever elected to the Legislative Assembly of Ontario, Canada, as a parliamentarian in 1990.

When I met my wife Rosalyn at Gallaudet, I quickly learned that her name sign was the same as mine, except she used the letter "R." As I took a liking to this young lady, I began to wonder if perhaps we weren't name-signed for each other!

Some of my school pals had very interesting name signs. One tall, skinny young lad wore pants that were always too big for him. He was forever reaching down and pulling them up. During a conversation he would be signing, his pants would begin to slip, and he would stop signing suddenly in mid-sentence, reach down, pull up his pants, and then resume the conversation. That visual distraction was about as bothersome to a deaf person as someone who repeatedly stopped to cough in mid-sentence would be to a hearing person. It is not surprising that this lad became known as "Pull-Up-Pants."

Another very small boy had the habit of sucking his thumb. The kids quickly dubbed him "Thumb Sucker," of course, and, just about as quickly as he arrived, he broke the habit. Unfortunately for the little fellow, and much to his dismay, the name sign stuck and lasted well into his high school years before it finally faded away and was replaced with "H-on-the-chin."

Another tall, broad-shouldered youth had two front teeth that were uneven. One was slightly longer than the other, and, I am sorry to say, "Long Tooth" became his name sign. No matter how hard the teachers and houseparents tried to abolish the sign, it persisted among his unthinking, insensitive young friends. It wasn't intended as an insult; they just thought it was a perfectly logical name sign. So when "Long Tooth," —I mean Tim, "T-on-the-chin," became a teenager he decided to take matters into his own hands. Coming from a very poor family, he got a job one summer, saved his money, and went to the dentist. The dentist did such a good job that it was hard to tell that one tooth had ever been longer than the other.

It took a while, however, to repair that old name sign habit. I remember that fall when Tim returned to school. He got off the chartered bus that brought all the kids from his section of the state to the MSD campus, beaming proudly, displaying his beautiful, new dental work behind an ear-to-ear grin. He stood there by the bus, hands in his pockets, just waiting for the kids to notice the difference. He really looked quite handsome. But kids, you know, don't always pay attention to such details. One of Tim's pals, noting Tim's arrival, ran up and greeted him. The pal pumped Tim's hand excitedly and inquired, "Hiya, Long Tooth, good summer?"

MR. ARONOVITZ AND US "WAYWARD DRUNKS"

Mr. Louis Aronovitz was an elderly, deaf houseparent in the intermediate department when I was an MSD student. His smile always warmed us. He was a friendly, articulate, and courteous gentleman from Kentucky. His name sign was an "A" on the forehead. He came to our school late in his career as he was nearing retirement. Mr. A had two noticeable and interesting characteristics: the way he smoked, and the way he walked—slowly, so as not to lose his balance.

He delighted in sharing the news of the day with his charges, and we grew up believing that he knew all the news in the world. Every day a bunch of us boys would gather around him in a semicircle and listen to him as he relayed what was happening in the world. But, to be honest, there was another reason we enjoyed watching him. Before he started, he'd always light up a cigarette, poke it in his mouth to free his hands for signing, take a few puffs then quickly forget about it, and move onto the news.

His cigarette would dangle from the corner of his mouth, à la Humphrey Bogart, and the smoke would curl upward, causing him to squint. As he signed, the ashes of that forgotten cigarette would get longer and longer, and we boys watched in suspense, glancing back and forth between the "news" and the lengthening ashes. Eventually, the ashes would fall and splatter on his suit lapel. He would look surprised, fingerspell and sign, "Ohhh, ohhh, excuse me" as if that was the first time it ever happened. He would quickly flick the ash-less cigarette, brush off his suit, put the cigarette back in his mouth, and forget about it again. Most of us boys agreed it would be much simpler to pause every now and then, take the cigarette out of the mouth and flick it, but who were we youngsters to tell an adult how to smoke?

Every Saturday afternoon was special. It was movie day at MSD. Back then, the movies cost twenty cents a person. We deaf kids paid only ten cents. (I always assumed they did not charge us for the sound.) Mr. Aronovitz would lead us small fries, two abreast, in a long line as we walked from the school campus to the movie house downtown. Because of his poor balance, he tended to stagger as he walked. He'd crisscross the sidewalk and, we in the line, thinking it was funny, did the same. Once in a while, when the sidewalk and the curb met, the sight of the curb depression caused him to lose his momentum, and he'd step down over the curb onto the edge of the street. Embarrassed, he would pretend he had moved there on purpose to check for stragglers, then he'd return to the head of the line and move on. If he wasn't looking, we too would march off the curb and back to the sidewalk. What a sight we must have been as we delightfully zigzagged our way to the movies behind Mr. A on a Saturday afternoon.

It is common knowledge in the Deaf community that many individuals lose their sense of balance when they become deaf, especially if they had a disease like spinal meningitis that causes a high fever. As young boys we did not know or understand this. As we grew older we learned why some of us had lost our balance and could not walk straight, just like Mr. A. We even teased each other about staggering like a drunk.

As I got older, what was once only a nighttime (walking in the dark) problem became just as bad (but more embarrassing) in broad daylight. When I am out walking in the field or along one of our trails, it has become almost impossible to walk a straight line. And that's when I think fondly of Mr. Aronovitz. Fortunately, I don't have a herd of boys, lined up two abreast, following me and giggling as I zigzag into old age. There's just the family dog sitting on her haunch, her ears perked, her head tilted sideways watching me and, no doubt, wondering where on earth I'm trying to go.

THE BROTHERS X

I was puzzled and surprised one hot, dry summer day when I looked up and saw a police car driving slowly up the road of Ten Rocky Acres leading a cloud of dust. The car stopped near the house and my friend, Russ Cochran, got out and approached me in the company of a police officer.

I had taught Russ sign language, and he was quite good at it. Russ signed that the officer wanted to know if I would be willing to come down to the city jail and talk with a deaf man who had been arrested for drunkenness. Russ told me he had tried to communicate with the man but had had no luck. The deaf man used different signs than I had taught him, Russ explained. It sounded like an adventure to me! I said sure immediately, and off we went to my first visit to jail. I was then about fourteen years old. Back then, interpreting wasn't yet a formal profession.

Downtown, I was ushered into the holding area of the city jail and stood outside one of the cells. Inside the cell was a tall, thin, unshaved man with long, uncombed hair. I didn't know him, but when I started signing to him, he became very excited. His face lit up, and a big grin quickly replaced his look of despair. I immediately saw why Russ could not understand the fellow. He used basic homemade signs and did not fingerspell at all. I realized I had to communicate with him through gestures. Instead of signing "policeman" and "drinking," I pointed to the policeman and imitated the act of drinking; for other information, I formed pictures in the air. When one concept did not work, I tried another and another until he understood. Through that process, we managed to communicate without too much difficulty.

I asked him his name, and instead of fingerspelling his name, he took out his billfold and showed me his driver's license. It was signed with an "X." That's when I realized he was illiterate, and that was why he did not fingerspell. He was the first illiterate deaf person I had ever met, and I was so startled to see the "X" signature that I cannot today remember his actual name. His license showed he was from a small neighboring town. With Russ interpreting, I learned from the police officer that "Mr. X" had been picked up for drunkenness the night before. The officer wanted me to tell Mr. X that it was against the law to get drunk within the city limits of West Plains and that the officer was willing to release him if he promised to get out of the city and stay out. For emphasis, the officer repeated "stay out" twice, shaking his finger at Mr. X in a scolding way.

I explained all this to Mr. X in what was a four-way conversation: the officer spoke to Russ and Russ signed to me, and I gestured to Mr. X. Mr. X then responded with gestures, which I verbally translated the best I could back to the officer. I did, however, feel a bit awkward about the whole situation. Here I was—a fourteen-year-old—standing outside a jail cell lecturing a forty-something-year-old on the other side of the bars.

Mr. X agreed to the officer's offer with a vigorous shake of his head. Satisfied with what he saw, the officer was only too happy to let the prisoner go. Everyone seemed happy and I returned to Ten Rocky Acres.

About a year later, my deaf friend, Frankie, took me to Bakersfield, a small neighboring town with a population of about 200, to meet some of his friends. To my surprise, Mr. X was one of them! He treated me like a hero, and, I suspect, he thought I was instrumental in springing him from jail. He introduced me to another man, who turned out to be his deaf brother who also had no name, and who I referred to as Mr. XX. I watched as Mr. X, using what seemed to be signs particular to their family, went through the motions of describing my visit with him at the city jail and telling Mr. XX how I had convinced his jailer to let him go. Mr. X put his arm around my shoulder and affectionately patted me, expressing his thanks and appreciation.

With Frankie's help and by repeatedly asking questions and picking up bits and pieces of information, I was able to put together some of the brothers' story. Both were in their late forties, and they made a living doing odd jobs for the townspeople. They appeared quite poor, wearing old, faded patched coveralls, tattered shirts, and sockless, ankle-high work shoes typical of the area. One of them pointed to an old, dilapidated house on a distant hill, and told me that that was where they lived. From Frankie, I learned that their parents were deceased and that they had inherited the family home. They were unmarried and had no immediate family members. In front of the house, parked on the incline, was their vintage car. It was parked facing downhill, the brothers explained, to guarantee that it would start. If the battery was low, they coasted down the hill and kicked in the clutch to get the engine going.

We spent the afternoon attending a local baseball game. Because of the brothers' illiteracy, there was little we could talk about in detail. It was interesting to watch how the brothers interacted with the townsfolk. Everyone seemed to know them and were courteous and friendly to the brothers. Many of the townsfolk communicated using common gestures. A hearing person would "talk" about how hot the weather was by wiping sweat from his forehead and shaking his head, and the brothers would imitate the gesture and wipe their foreheads and nod their heads in agreement to indicate that they understood. The hearing person would point to Frankie and me and give us an A-OK gesture and shake our hands, to say they were pleased to meet the brothers' friends. It was obvious that the brothers were well-known and even well-liked. They also appeared to be the town's adopted mascots, since Frankie and I observed that they were treated more like children than adults. The small-town atmosphere seemed quite appropriate for their situation.

Following the baseball game, which was the town's big event, we stopped by a local café to get something to eat. Frankie and I read the menu and placed our orders. Since the two brothers couldn't read, I watched to see how they would order what they wanted. Naturally, they had no use for the menu. They looked at the waitress, who obviously knew them, and ordered using gestures. In this case, one of them fanned his hand in front of his mouth indicating hot, then cupped both hands in the shape of a bowl and placed the bowl on the table, and went through the motion of eating from the bowl with an imaginary spoon. The waitress quickly nodded her head that she understood, wrote down the order, and left. I sat there amazed. It was as quick as that! Their bowls of soup arrived with the sandwiches Frankie and I had ordered. I did wonder later what they did if they wanted a particular kind of soup.

As we paid for our lunches, the brothers simply handed the waitress a pile of dollar bills. She picked out the correct amount, gave them some change, and returned the rest.

On the way home that afternoon, Frankie and I talked about the brothers. Frankie said that their parents had known about the deaf school, but had refused to send their sons away. As young boys, they had been placed in the local public school, but obviously, it had not worked for them. What disturbed Frankie and me the most was the knowledge that none of this had to happen. These two deaf persons could have had access to an education but were denied because of their parents' refusal to face the reality of their sons being deaf. As a result, the brothers were destined to lives of ignorance and poverty and denied the opportunity to achieve their fullest potential. More than any other incident in my life, this sad experience taught me the importance of education.

My mother and I were very close. She was a very gentle, sensitive, caring woman. During the summertime, we often spent hours sitting at the kitchen table just talking. One day, weeks after the Bakersfield trip, I told Mom about the experience and how shocked I was to learn that the X brothers' parents had not been willing to send them away to school. That was when I learned about the trauma my parents had endured in making a similar decision about my education. They, too, had been confronted with the decision of placing me in the local public school or sending me away from home to the residential school for deaf children, a decision they found very hard to make. My mother told me how some relatives, especially my grandmother, were adamantly opposed to the idea of sending me away. She had spent many agonizing hours over the decision that first year I was away, wondering if what she had done was right.

I admitted to Mom something I had never told anyone else, that there were times when I, too, got lonesome and homesick

Pop, my grandfather, and me prior to going to Gallaudet College in 1954.

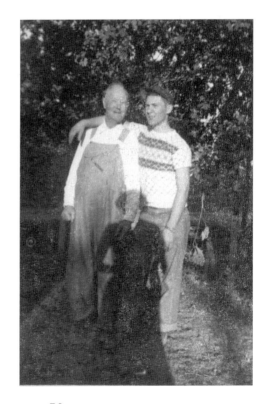

and missed the family. But I told her how much I enjoyed school, my classmates, my teachers, and being in an environment where I was not constantly running into limiting, frustrating communication barriers. And where I had so many opportunities to learn and grow and, most importantly, the freedom to be myself. Mom nodded her head, smiled as she gently placed her hand on mine, and looked me in the eyes, "Jack, I know. Dad and I are so glad we made that choice."

I nodded, "Mom, so am I. So am I."

MR. ARNOVITZ'S GIRLFRIEND

Mr. Arnovitz, our houseparent, had an elderly deaf lady friend who us boys liked to tease him was his girlfriend. She was one of the girls' houseparents, so Mr. Arnovitz and the lady often chatted in the school dining room when the boys and girls got together for meals.

Mr. Arnovitz liked to tell us the story about his lady friend and her hat. He recalled the time she bought a pretty new hat with long, beautiful feathers sticking out the top. One day she went shopping downtown and passed a store that caught her fancy. She went inside to browse around, and while checking some merchandise on a low counter, she bent over for a closer look. Unbeknownst to her, one of the long feathers on her hat touched a lighted candle on a shelf above. As she straightened up, a store clerk noticed the feather was on fire and yelled at her, but being deaf, she did not hear the warning and strolled on. The clerk shouted again in vain before suddenly realizing that the woman was deaf and ran up to her, yanked the hat off her head, threw it on the floor, and stomped out the blaze. Mr. Arnovitz's lady friend was alarmed at such rudeness of her new hat being stomped to pieces on the floor until she realized what had happened.

Mr. Arnovitz always squinted his eyes and did a belly chuckle when he told the story. We boys enjoyed it, too, but we still thought the story about Mr. Arnovitz's arrest, which we had heard from another houseparent, was funnier. It happened one evening when Mr. Arnovitz was off duty. He decided to walk downtown to the Spot Café, a popular local eatery, for a late-night snack. It was very dark when he set out on his return to the campus. To make matters worse, he had to pass through an area that was poorly lit. As usual, he had difficulty keeping his balance in the dark, and staying on the sidewalk. His stagger got so bad that a new city policeman driving by on his patrol took notice. The policeman decided to drive around the block and check again.

Convinced he had a drunk on his hands, the policeman turned on his flashing lights and stopped Mr. Arnovitz. The officer was in the process of arresting him when Mr. Arnovitz took out his pad and pencil and explained what the problem was. He was very embarrassed, but the young officer observed how well he wrote. Since Mr. Arnovitz was putting up such a heated argument, the officer consented to drive him to the campus and talk with the school superintendent.

The superintendent thanked the officer for giving Mr. Arnovitz a ride and explained the difficulty some deaf people experience with their balance, especially when it is dark. The superintendent assured the young man that it was definitely not a bottle of spirits that was the cause of Mr. Arnovitz's stagger.

TIME AND THE REVEREND WESTERTHAM

The Reverend Westertham was a fire-and-brimstone preacher. He was a tall, thin man with a thick shock of wavy silver hair that topped his long, narrow, reddish face. Piercing eyes darted above his long, pointed nose on which perched a pair of round, steel-framed glasses.

Reverend Westertham was a hearing man who, as a young fella, befriended a neighborhood deaf boy. As a result of this encounter, he felt the call to ministry and chose to perform deaf missionary work. Because of the scarcity of deaf congregations, his work took him to several states, and he always made it a practice to stop and preach at schools for the deaf when he was in their areas. MSD was one of them.

Rosalyn saw him at the North Carolina School for the Deaf and has no idea what his voice sounded like, but if it in any way resembled his signs and facial expressions, it surely must have been a powerful one. When he got warmed up in the process of delivering one of his fiery sermons, his face turned a certain shade of red, and his eyes took on a stern, penetrating look. Sitting in the crowded audience, you got the feeling that those eyes could see right through you, and you were immediately sorry if you had done anything wrong in the past week because you were sure he knew what it was. Rosalyn remembers how she used to squirm when he preached to us students at Sunday assembly. If you had been naughty the previous week, you sure wanted God's forgiveness quickly—not so much because of what you had done wrong, but because of your fear that Reverend Westertham would find out. With his thundering voice, as I imagined it, his red face, his fierce facial expressions, and his powerful signs that seemed to shake the stage he stood on, I am sure that even the devil would not have wanted to get too close to him.

It was in January, after Christmas, when all that changed. On that particular day, Reverend Westertham was in the middle of one of his heated sermons. He was warning the audience about the consequences of sin.

"Sinners go to hell!" he thundered, pounding his clenched fist on the podium, sending vibrations that could be felt in the front rows.

IF YOU . . . , he signed, pointing to each person in the audience in a wide, sweeping arch. He was so worked up that when he signed YOU swiftly and forcefully, his new gold wristwatch, which he had just received for Christmas, slid off his wrist and went flying into the middle of the auditorium. It shattered into pieces when it crashed on the floor.

A classmate poked me in the arm with his elbow. "Even time can't keep up with Reverend Westertham," he signed to me.

"HEY KID! YOU DEAF OR SOMETHING?!"

We had only one family car, which Dad drove to work every day. If my siblings and I wanted to go to town or someplace, we walked. When I was fifteen years old, my parents finally let me ride my brother's hand-me-down bicycle to town. They had withheld permission as long as they could, I knew, because I was deaf. After seeing all the freedom my hearing friends had on their bicycles, some who were much younger than me, I had rebelled, and my parents had reluctantly and grudgingly given in. I cherished the new freedom the bicycle gave me in the same way my son and daughter, years later, cherished the liberty our family vehicle gave them when they turned sixteen.

One day I was returning home from a trip downtown on the bicycle when I decided to take a short cut, which went over a steep, narrow hill. I was pedaling the bike up a steep, narrow, one-lane street when I became very tired, and about halfway up the hill, I stopped to rest and catch my breath.

It didn't seem very long after I had stopped when I noticed people glancing my way. My "deaf sense" immediately told me something was wrong. I quickly turned around, and sure enough, there was a long line of cars behind me. It was obvious that the drivers had been honking and honking, trying to tell me to get out of the way! Mortified, I quickly pulled the bike over to the side of the road and let the cars pass.

I stood there as calmly as I could, a feeble smile on my face, and watched the cars go by. The occupants of each car stared at me sternly with cold, quizzical looks, and on each face was written the same visual message: "Hey, what's the matter with you kid, you deaf or something?!"

DAD

My father was Floyd Lester Gannon. He came from a large, poor family of eight brothers and sisters. His father had died when Dad was about five years old, and so he would later drop out of school in the third grade to help support the family. Dad had very little formal schooling, but he was a graduate of the "school of hard knocks." He was a hard worker who piled rocks and cut sprouts—back-breaking work. This outdoor work gave him a strong body, stamina, and a permanent tan.

Dad learned to grease and service cars when he was young, and he spent most of his working life in garages and at gas stations where he earned the nickname "Shorty" because of his short stature. He called himself a grease monkey, a trade I had thought of pursuing when I was a youngster. In many ways, Dad's hands were a reflection of his life. He had short, stocky, scarred hands toughened from years of manual labor and cracked grease-stained fingernails.

At home, Dad loved working around Ten Rocky Acres. He never lost his love for the outdoors, a love that he passed on to me. He raised hogs and chickens, and we had a horse. He was always fixing fences, installing fence posts in the rocky soil, and cutting and piling brush. As a country boy, I learned the value of a pocketknife. This formed another link between the two of us. Dad thought it unthinkable not to have a pocketknife, and he made sure I always had one, and I have carried one all my life. He and I would work side-by-side for hours without hardly uttering a word, an activity that formed a bond between the two of us that is hard to describe even today.

As a hard worker, Dad expected the same from others. If he caught me being idle, he would quickly find something for me to do. After I became a white-collar professional, he asked me to explain what I did. So I told him about my work and mentioned the trips I took and the talks I gave. He looked at me, only half-kidding, and said, "You mean they pay you to talk?!" He could never figure out how "giving a talk" could be considered work.

The name "Ten Rocky Acres" was no exaggeration. It was a patch of earth covered in millions of rocks. I always believed we owned the rockiest patch on earth. If there was any rich, loamy soil on the property, I never found it. But Dad loved those rocks, and the family joke was that if you took one, you'd better get his permission or risk his reaction. He would pick up the unusual, pretty rocks and use them to line a flower bed or put on display.

He used the "undesirables" with his concrete mix or piled them on a slope to level off the ground or for shoring up a rock wall. One summer, after I was married and our children were young, we paid my parents a visit. Dad and our daughter, Christy, who was very small, went out "looking for rocks." Now a grown lady, she still has those pretty rocks she and her grandpa collected that summer.

Dad had his own special brand of homespun humor. One day I was eating an apple and discovered a worm in it. Shocked, I gasped, "Dad! Look! There's a worm in my apple!" He took a casual look and said, "Don't worry, Jack, it won't eat much."

One summer, we acquired a pretty, brown horse with white markings. It was during the era when automobile manufacturers were breaking away from the long tradition of turning out only black cars and had begun producing cars in two colors. These cars were popularly referred to as two tones. Dad named our new horse "Tutone."

Another time, we had a big, red sow Dad named "Suzie" after a neighborhood girl with the same color of hair. Dad told me that the sow didn't seem to mind, but Suzie, the neighbor, wasn't very happy about sharing her name with the sow.

Money was scarce all of Dad's life, and so he was very frugal. It was difficult to get him to part with one of his hard-earned dollars unless it had something to do with fishing gear. He loved to fish and so was a bit more generous in that area. Dad always bought second-hand cars on installment plans. I once asked him why he didn't buy a new car. "'Cause," he said, "they ain't worth it." End of discussion.

Because of his frugal habits he would collect and save almost everything—scrap iron, old furniture, discarded lumber, etc. When one of his employees decided to get rid of some junk cars, Dad volunteered to tow them to Ten Rocky Acres. Apparently he had visions of turning the place into a salvage lot and "getting rich," much to the family's dismay. It was years before we finally got rid of those old cars.

At the garage where he worked, after changing a car's oil and before discarding the can, he would turn it upside down and let the last few drops drip into a large oil can. After a period of time, he brought home a barrel almost full of those "oil drips."

Dad was not a very organized person. He did not have a place to put all his tools, nor the habit of putting them where they belonged. Instead, he left them where he was last working on a project. When I asked where a pick or shovel was, he would stop and think a moment before saying, "Look over near the corner fence," "Look behind the woodpile," or "Down by the pond." When I stop and look at my paper-cluttered desk, I think about what else I inherited from him.

Being deaf, of course, had its benefits, especially when Dad got angry or upset and started swearing. Boy, could he swear! He would let out a stream of profanity—sorry, none of it printable—that could burn the bark off a tree. Deadeye, our dog, and I would cower nearby, and I would squint my eyes—so as not to "hear" too much—until the thunder passed. I'm happy to say this is one thing I didn't inherit from him.

Dad was a very strict disciplinarian. He made known with his hand or belt what he considered right or wrong, and there was no room for argument. To him, arguing was a form of disrespect. He was a man who did not know how to share his inner feelings or thoughts. It made him feel awkward and embarrassed. That was one reason I grew up with the impression that expressing affection for others was not an accepted practice and, definitely, not "manly." The only time I saw Dad cry was at Grandma's funeral. I still remember the shock I felt that day: my father could cry.

Likewise, he did not know how to express love. I do not ever remember him kissing me, and am quite vague about whether or not I ever got a hug. I knew he loved me, but he did not know how to express love openly.

He and I discussed my being deaf only once. That day, I complained to him that I did not like being deaf. I complained about the embarrassment I felt when a person talked to me behind my back or when I could not understand what was being said. I complained about how frustrating it was to carry on a limited spoken conversation and often not knowing what the family was talking about. I told him I wanted to hear like the rest of the family. Dad listened in silence, nodding now and then to acknowledge my words. As soon as I was through with my tirade, he shrugged his shoulders, looked at me in earnest, put his hand on my shoulder, and said in his matter-of-fact way, "Jack, that's the way you are."

At first, I was miffed by his abrupt, insensitive response but gradually I came to understand what he meant. He was telling me to accept what life had handed me and make the most of it. His life was an example. In that simple response, he planted a seed of acceptance of who I was that gave root to a philosophy that has not only helped me accept being deaf, but in many ways has helped me to see it as the blessing in disguise that it is. Accepting myself as I was and making the best of it was the most important lesson Dad ever taught me.

I was a father of two children of my own when I finally managed to tell Dad how I felt about him one summer. I had married into a very loving family. Rosalyn's family was always very generous with their affection, and it had rubbed off on me. Thanks to Rosalyn, our own family became a hugging, kissing, love-expressing family. We had come for a visit that summer, and it was now time to return home. When we traveled, we liked to get up very early in the morning and get on the road. When we were ready to leave, I went into Dad's bedroom to tell him goodbye. He was still in bed; he hadn't been feeling well. Emphysema, from long years of smoking, had begun to take its toll, and he often had to rely on an oxygen tank to breathe.

I gently woke him, reached down and hugged him, and said, "I love you, Dad." Dad looked up at me silently, smiled, nodded his head, and to my surprise, responded, "I love you, too." It was the first time in our lives we had ever said that to each other. I left the room blurry-eyed and deeply touched from the exchange. I would be forever grateful it happened because the following December, Dad was gone.

At his funeral, I took out my pocketknife and placed it in his hand to be buried with him.

MY FRIEND, WILLIE, THE BOOTBLACK

Willie was an African American bootblack in my hometown in the Ozark mountains. During the summer, when I was home from school, I often stopped by the barbershop in the town square, where he shined shoes. He always seemed delighted to see me. Willie and I had a common bond; we were both deaf.

Willie must have been in his late sixties the first time I met him. He was tall and lanky with stooped shoulders and long, bony fingers with large knuckles. A crown of black-and-white fuzz ringed his bald head. It looked like someone had sprinkled salt and pepper on it. Gold-capped teeth glistened in his mouth whenever he flashed his ear-to-ear grin, which was often because he was a happy person.

Willie could not speak and that was why the town folks called him "Dummy." By the clientele he attracted, however, it was obvious that many of the local businessmen considered him the best bootblack in town. Willie took great pride in his work and had a knack for pleasing his customers. He earned twenty cents a shoeshine. When he was busy with a customer, I sat and watched him work. He went through a familiar routine, which included an imaginary dance act that always amused his customers. He displayed rhythm that looked like he was listening to music, but, of course, he wasn't. After applying polish to both shoes, he would take out his buffer cloth, hold it in both hands high above his head—somewhat like a pitcher winding up for a pitch—bend his body a little bit, then hit the shoes with gusto and rapid motion. Soon he had a sparkle glinting from each shoe. Then, when he was through, he would take a low bow—like an actor on a stage—to signal that the job was done. And, as the customer climbed down from the high shoeshine chair, Willie never missed the opportunity to straighten the customer's collar or brush off his jacket or pamper him in some other way. In the process, he always turned and cast a sly wink at me to tell me to watch the results. It seldom failed to earn him a hefty tip!

Although I am ashamed to admit it now, I never learned Willie's full name. Nor did I ever learn much about his background, his family, or his education. I only knew he lived in a boarding house, and it was clear that he had received very little schooling. Most segregated schools for Black deaf children during those times were drastically underfunded.

Even so, Willie had a lot of common sense and a fairly good grasp of sign language, so we never had any trouble communicating with each other. He had one amusing quirk. He loved to tell me how "rich" he was. I always thought he had a wild, wishful imagination because every time he started talking about how much money he had, the sum had grown to another exorbitant amount! Gradually, I learned that Willie was rich in another way. He was rich in spirit and pride.

As a youth during those early years, I was easily embarrassed by being deaf. While I had understandable speech, my lipreading skills were only fair. When someone spoke to me and I did not understand, I quickly became flustered. With all the emphasis on oralism that was prevalent during my school days, I had developed the feeling that I was a failure as a lipreader and that this failure and my deafness were an *imposition* on hearing people, and I was to blame for this.

One day it suddenly occurred to me that if I thought I had it bad, Willie was in a much worse situation than me—he could neither read, write, speak, nor lipread. He communicated with everyone by gesture and by vigorously nodding or shaking his head. At first, I was a little embarrassed by Willie's style, but I noticed he did not let his inability to understand everything people said faze him one little bit. If he didn't understand someone, he just shrugged his bony shoulders and shook his head. One day, I asked him about that after a customer, who had spoken to him, left. I doubted he had fully understood what the customer had said.

Instead of answering my query directly, he just shrugged his shoulders and pointed his index finger at me and then at himself and signed, YOU, ME, then pointing at the hearing people around the barber shop, DIFFERENT. Then he told me how proud he was of his job and the work he did. "My shine's the best!" he said. He pointed his long finger at me again and waving it in a scolding manner he signed sternly, "You always be proud of yourself!"

That is one piece of advice I have never forgotten.

At the end of the day, while waiting for Mom to finish her work at the nearby shoe store and take me home, I watched Willie sweep the barbershop with his long push broom and then put away his shoe shine equipment. He would button up his aged blue pinstriped vest, don his jacket and hat, get his cane, wave goodbye to me and his coworkers, and head for home. He'd head down North Main toward the section of the town where all the Black people lived. I'd smile as I watched him go. Even though to many, he was "deaf, mute, Black, and illiterate," to me, he was the perfect image of a proud, successful businessman going home after a day's work.

Many years later, during my work at Gallaudet University, I attended a workshop on alumni and public relations, one of my areas of responsibility. The consultant who was leading the session told the story about the time he was asked what he would like to see engraved on his tombstone. What a strange, bizarre question to ask someone, I thought. The consultant, whose job involved working with alumni and public relations personnel at colleges, universities, corporations, and organizations throughout the nation, told us how he had responded to that question.

"Four words," he said. "I'd like to see my tombstone read: 'He made a difference.'"

His comments immediately reminded me of Willie. I saw again that tall, thin, old man with his gold teeth and salt-and-pepper hair stooping over me and shaking his long bony index finger in a scolding manner and telling me, PROUD SELF ALWAYS! We can only be proud of ourselves by taking pride in what we do and by what we achieve and by making a difference.

I have shared this story with many deaf young people I have talked with in my travels around the nation. I tell them about Willie, and the sage advice this supposedly "illiterate" man had given me so many years ago when I was a little boy. I use the story to remind young people that it is all right to be who they are, and I challenge them to get all the education they can and use it—and their lives—to make a difference in the world in which they live.

AND, SHE HAD RED HAIR

I felt a breeze and a bundle of energy coming into the class-room the day I first noticed her. What caught my attention was her cheerfulness; she was the happiest person I had ever laid eyes on. And I thought she was quite pretty, too. There was only one thing I was not sure about: she had red hair. After being teased without mercy about being interested in a redhead when I was in the second grade, I never again glanced twice at a girl with red hair. But something was different about Rosalyn Faye Lee, and I could not take my eyes off her.

A graduate of the North Carolina School for the Deaf in Morganton, Rosalyn became deaf from mastoid fever when she was eighteen months old. An art major at Gallaudet, she was also on the swimming and field hockey teams, and later served as president of her sorority. As I gradually got to know her better, I found a rare, independent-minded, sensitive, thoughtful, and caring individual. The smile she always wore reflected a person-ality that was as warm and natural as sunshine. Almost over-night, love made me color-blind; I no longer noticed her red hair. It took me forever, but one day, I finally managed to build up enough courage to ask her for a date.

Almost everyone else had gone to a campus-wide event, except for Rosalyn and a few classmates who were working in Chapel Hall, preparing for our upcoming prep class play. I was delighted to find her there. She was perched high on a ladder painting backdrops. Although I waved at her to get her attention, I could not get her to look my way. I tapped on the ladder, but she still didn't feel a thing. I shook the ladder gently to get her attention. She jumped, and signed, STOP THAT! FINISH! Startled and perhaps scared, she glared down at me.

She wondered why I wasn't at the other event, and why I was bothering her when she was so busy. As I looked up at her nervously, she made it very clear that she did not like my shaking the ladder. I asked her for a date. To my relief, she consented to the date and agreed to accompany me to a carnival hosted by a fraternity.

The date turned out to be only half a date, but at least it was a start. Caught sneaking out of the dorm during study hour to run to the corner store for snacks for her roommates, Rosalyn received a month's suspension. After much pleading, the dean granted her permission to attend part of the carnival. That first date would change my life, and we courted throughout college.

Our closeness, love, and respect for each other grew. I still have never gotten over how lucky I am.

The day our prep year came to a close, students began to leave the campus. Sterling, my roommate, found me and told me the inevitable: "Mr. Lee wants to meet you." That was the summons I had been dreading. With butterflies churning in my stomach, I went to meet Rosalyn's parents for the first time. I don't exaggerate when I say that Mr. Lee looked like a giant. I looked up at the six-foot-four towering figure, who was wearing old-fashioned round, wire-framed glasses. Suddenly I wished I was somewhere else. I said, "Hi."

Myself and my girlfriend, Rosalyn, at the Junior/Senior Prom, 1956.

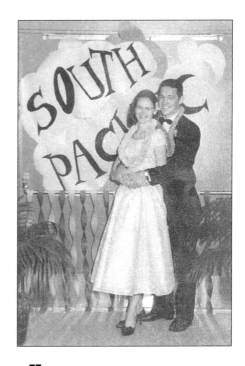

To my surprise, Mr. Lee greeted me warmly, holding out a big hand. As we shook hands, I felt as if his went around mine twice. I didn't know it then, of course, but Mr. Lee and I would become very good friends. He became a second father and a person for whom I had much affection.

When I turned to greet Rosalyn's mother, I immediately realized I was looking at a warm, friendly, carbon copy of the girl I knew. I quickly felt at ease.

Rosalyn had three sisters. Her oldest, Nancy, had already left home. Rosalyn and her two younger hearing sisters, Sara Ann

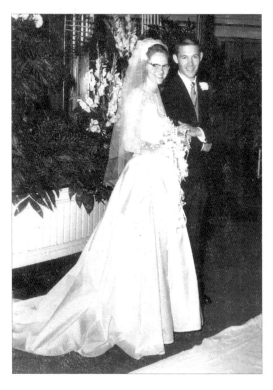

We got married five days after our graduation in 1959.

and Martha, had developed their own form of homemade signs as some families with a deaf member do. Even after Rosalyn went away to school and began learning American Sign Language (ASL), the sisters continued to use home signs. Whenever home from school, Rosalyn reverted to using their home signs.

When I watched the three sisters signing, I felt like I was witnessing deaf foreigners. I could not understand what they were saying, so Rosalyn had to interpret for me. It was then that Rosalyn's sisters learned that they had been using homemade signs rather than sign language.

The Lee sisters were horse fanatics. They rode, trained, and jumped horses and participated in horse shows all over the state. Rosalyn once had second thoughts about participating in a horse show because she could not hear the judge's commands for routines, but her father would not let her use this as an excuse. Instead, Rosalyn's sisters stood outside the ring where she could see them and signed any changes in routine, and she did it just fine.

Five days after we graduated from college in 1959, Rosalyn and I married in North Carolina. My mother and younger brother Don rode the bus from Missouri to Washington, DC, for commencement and then attended the wedding; Don was my best man. Many of our classmates also attended. Interpreting the ceremony was Ed Scouten, the dean and professor of the preparatory class who so patiently stood at the entrance of

Drake House during our prep year, holding the door open for me countless times. As I passed the threshold into the building, he always looked up at the clock on the wall to be sure I had arrived on time.

Newlyweds, Rosalyn and I began our teaching careers that fall at the Nebraska School for the Deaf (NSD) in Omaha. I'm glad she forgave me for shaking the ladder.

THE ALASKAN OLD-TIMER

The summer following our sophomore year at Gallaudet College, my college classmates Bill Sugiyama, Vilas Johnson, and I purchased and drove an old pickup truck to Alaska in search of adventure. We were very fortunate to secure summer employment on the grounds crew at the University of Alaska in the town of College, about five miles north of Fairbanks. That summer the university was undergoing quite a bit of construction, and we were hired to help landscape the grounds and plant grass. That's where we came into contact with the "Old-Timer."

My classmates, Vilas Johnson and Bill Sugiyama, and me in Alaska, 1957.

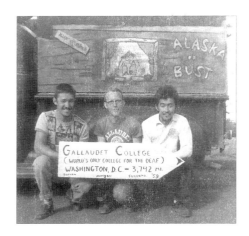

81

We called him the "Old-Timer" because we never learned his real name. The day we met the Old-Timer, we saw him slowly, cautiously, hobbling down the stairs from the second-floor cafeteria of the Student Union Building at the University of Alaska. Bill, Vilas, and I had just finished our lunch and, as usual, we sat in the lounge area near the door, resting, chatting, and watching people pass. We casually observed the Old-Timer as he came down the steps. We had seen him limp by many times before, and we had always wondered why he walked so slowly and cautiously. It looked as if his feet hurt and that he was afraid of falling. We had also noticed that all the fingers on both his hands were missing except for his thumbs and pinky fingers. He was, we were sure, aware that we were deaf because we had seen him watching us sign to each other.

On this particular day, as we sat in the lounge, he surprised us by stopping directly in front of where we were. His aged, watery eyes looked at each of us intently. He didn't say a word. He then looked down at his feet and, with the heel of one foot behind the heel of the other, pushed off one of his slippers, and lifted his leg, and held up what remained of his foot merely inches from my face.

Bill and Vilas and I were stunned. What we saw was only half a foot. Pink, tender skin covered the front of the foot where toes had once been. We looked at the grisly sight, then at each other, shaking our heads slowly in disbelief. We swallowed in unison and attempted feeble smiles as we looked up at him and nodded in acknowledgment. We were not sure what he was trying to tell us, but our nodding told him we understood. Satisfied, he slipped the stump back into the slipper, then with the thumb of one hand, pointed first at us then at himself, winked, nodded, smiled, turned around precariously, and slowly hobbled out the door.

The three of us looked at one another again, puzzled. It eventually dawned on us that he was probably trying to tell us that all four of us had something in common. We were four disabled brothers. Naturally, the discovery of the Old-Timer's foot and finger amputations bothered us and aroused our curiosity, and we inquired among our coworkers what had happened. We learned that the Old-Timer was an alcoholic. On a very cold, Alaska winter night, we were told, the drunk Old-Timer was on his way home from a local bar when he stumbled, rolled off the sidewalk, and fell asleep. By the time he was found, his fingers and toes had frozen and had to be amputated.

Some days later, after that "introduction" in the Student Union, Vilas and I were working by the president's residence near the end of the huge campus. In the distance, we could see the Old-Timer watering the flowers and rose bushes around the house.

Later, the Old-Timer approached us and began talking. Neither Vilas nor I could understand what he was trying to say, and we shook our heads, but he would not give up. He pointed his hand in the direction of the house and uttered something again and again. By his behavior and insistency, we knew he was asking for something but could not figure out what it was. Both Vilas and I always carried a pad and pen for such situations, and we reached for them but stopped in mid-motion when we saw his hands and realized he could not hold a pen and write.

He pointed a thumb to his lips and spoke again. He was so difficult to lipread neither of us could fathom what he was trying to say. I nudged Vilas aside and tried alone. I looked intently at his lips and asked him to repeat what he had said. He spoke again, but again, I did not understand him. I turned to Vilas and signed: "What did he say?" Vilas shrugged. He didn't know either.

Then Vilas tried. He held up the flattened palms of his hands, hunched his shoulders and gestured, "What?" while watching the Old-Timer's lips closely. The Old-Timer spoke again and Vilas turned to me and signed: "What did he say?" We both knew he wanted something, but we still could not figure out what it was. If only he would point to something, or gesture, or give us some clue. He stood there with despair etched on his face, repeating himself over and over, and waving his hands in circles in the air.

All three of us felt frustrated. A feeling of helplessness crept over Vilas and me. We desperately wanted to understand and to help, but we had no idea what he wanted.

I tried once more. This time I bent over, put my hands on my knees to steady my gaze, squinted my eyes to get the best possible focus, and concentrated with all my might on his lips. Feeling a bit better prepared for the challenge this time, I hastily said, "What?" and stared at his lips.

The Old-Timer took my cue. He, too, leaned forward and put his hands on my shoulders to steady himself. He positioned his nose inches from mine, then he wrinkled his deeply furrowed brow, raised his eyebrows in an attempt to straighten up his face, and once more repeated himself, this time much slower than before. As he opened his mouth, my nostrils caught a strong whiff of the chewing tobacco and alcohol on his breath.

Instead of catching that elusive bit of spoken information, as I had hoped, I saw only a pair of sad, watery eyes looking at me in despair and a couple days' growth of stubble on his weathered, unshaven face. His thinning gray hair waved in the morning breeze, and tobacco spittle streaked down the corners of his mouth. I also noted, for the first time, that many of his teeth were missing. The remaining teeth were crooked and to-bacco-stained.

I could see that the Old-Timer was making a greater effort to be understood. He opened his mouth wider, thinking that he was speaking clearer, but unfortunately, that only distracted me further because I then saw a wad of chewing tobacco dancing around on his tongue. There was simply no way I could ignore all the distractions and concentrate on what he was trying to tell me.

We were on the verge of giving up entirely when a young hearing coworker happened by. An "I've-been-saved" look of relief swept over the Old-Timer's face when he looked up and saw the young man. The Old-Timer and I straightened up. He smiled at the newcomer and spoke a few words. Vilas and I looked at the young fellow, saw him nod his head, smile and say, "Oh, sure!" Vilas and I then watched the two of them return to where the Old-Timer had been working and saw the young fellow unscrew the garden hose and take it to the other side of the house and hook it up. So that was what the Old-Timer had been trying to ask us to do!

Vilas and I looked at each other with "I've-never-felt-so-dumb" expressions on our faces. We felt humiliated and disappointed at not being able to help, which we would have gladly done. But we had been deaf long enough to know that such incidents happen and that there was nothing we could do about them. We realized that, as usual, we on the deaf end of the conversation were getting blamed for the communication failure. As usual, people who talk don't realize that spoken communication is a two-way street—sending and receiving—and when one part doesn't succeed, the communication breaks down. Both sides—the sender and the receiver—have a responsibility to see that the conversation succeeds. Often deaf people are better than hearing people at making themselves understood, even when they have to gesture or point.

Lipreading classes had yet to teach me how to lipread tobacco-stained lips or a mouth full of missing and broken teeth. We shrugged and went back to work.

RON MEETS HIS FUTURE MOTHER-IN-LAW

Ron, a Gallaudet College student, had planned his trip so that he could stop by and see his sweetheart on his way to a summer job in another state. He arrived in her hometown, located her house, and nervously rang the doorbell.

As he waited, he experienced the anxiety every suitor feels when meeting a girlfriend's (or boyfriend's) parents for the first time. A middle-aged woman came to the door and opened it. Ron, who was born deaf and had no speech skills, quickly handed her a note he had written in advance. "Does Melvia live here?" the note asked. "Is she home?"

The woman, who turned out to be Melvia's mother, read the note and shook her head negatively. She picked up a pencil from a table near the door and wrote, "No. She is out, but she will be back soon."

A look of disappointment crept over Ron's face as he read the response. Noticing the disappointment, the lady invited Ron into the house to wait for Melvia. For the next hour or so, they carried on a conversation by writing notes back and forth. At long last, Melvia returned home, and seeing Ron, her face brightened into a happy smile and she rushed into his outstretched arms.

After a long embrace, Melvia stepped back and introduced Ron to her mother in sign language. Dumbstruck, Ron looked at Melvia's mother then at Melvia. "She knows sign language?!" he inquired. Almost simultaneously, Melvia's mother exclaimed, "He knows sign language?!"

"Of course, you both know sign language!" signed a surprised Melvia. "You're both deaf!" Suddenly it occurred to Melvia that she had neglected to tell Ron and her mother that they all were deaf. They had spent a couple hours writing back and forth when, naturally, they could have simply carried on a more comfortable conversation by signing to each other.

PART TWO

BECOMING TEACHERS AND COACHES

words from a deaf child

I need to perceive life through native eyes
not yours, which after all, are yours.
you're sailing on a vastly foreign sea
it's my country—you're the stranger
listen to me.

we sign a language all our own
our hands are yours to share
the word, I think, is communication
and more than that, communion,
we speak through sign and both together
whatever and by all the means to the end.

millions of stars do not make me a star
millions of dreams may not be my dream
the pilgrims were a handful on a newfound shore
that was their own.

let me choose if I will
to be different from the mass
learn that there is beauty in a single star
peace and grace in being what you are.

like an almighty wave this flash of scorn
for you who do not try to understand

that every sunset, every sunrise born

is different as each single grain of sand.

this life is yours to know but mine to command

teach me, love me, like you'd love a work of art

or a mountain pine

don't try to lead me, own me, force me

into a mold that's not my own.

water, feed, nourish the growing tree

don't hold it, fold it, circumscribe

let it flower, let it grow

if you love me, let me go.

—Mervin D. Garretson

Mervin D. Garretson (1923–2013) grew up in a large family on a Wyoming ranch, most likely with his nose in a book. He and his pals often rode their bikes thirteen miles to the next town to get books from the library. He was one of the earliest deaf principals of a school for the deaf during his time, an educator, a leader's leader, and a strong, logical Deaf individual. He was the author of two books.

INTRODUCTION

In 1954, Jack enrolled in Gallaudet to earn a bachelor of science degree in education. Back then, Gallaudet College (now University) was a small, selective college with an enrollment of 294. By 1959, this grew to 383 when Jack graduated along with his college sweetheart Rosalyn Faye Lee. Commencement and their marriage ceremony were separated by only five days, and the newlyweds moved to Nebraska, where both began teaching careers at NSD. Jack taught printing, graphic arts, and photography, while Rosalyn taught art and physical education. Jack continued taking graduate courses at Omaha University and Ball State University. In Omaha, Jack coached the basketball and football teams at NSD. He was president of the Omaha Club of the Deaf and also coached the club's basketball team. At the state level, Jack served as president of the Nebraska Association of the Deaf. After nine years in Nebraska, the Gannons returned to Washington, DC, where Jack began working for Gallaudet.

"...AS THE TWIG IS BENT..."

I stood in the doorway of the printshop at NSD's vocational building and looked into the room. This was the room that would be the center of my life for the next several years. Here, I would introduce my young deaf students to the creative world of printing and help prepare them for the world of work. I would teach them typesetting, press and bindery work, film and print-making, lithography, and as much of that "foreign" language called English as I could. From that moment on, I always felt the weight of responsibility for each student's future.

The room's dirty yellowish brick walls looked like they had never been painted. In the far corner sat a huge, oily, old hand-fed Babcock newspaper press. Rows of type cabinets with their California job cases full of type stood next to two makeup tables. Two long wooden printers' tables sat near the center of the room for folding the school's publications and other print jobs. Next to them was an attractive old rolltop desk for the teacher, piled high with papers—letters, galley proofs, paper catalogs, and job tickets. Along one wall were three turn-of-the-century hand-fed platen presses of different sizes. Near another wall was a Kluge automatic platen press. It appeared to be about twenty years old and was probably the newest piece of equipment in the shop. I felt I was looking more at a printshop museum than at a modern classroom. The dismal sight that greeted my eyes that moment was not encouraging and made me wonder if I had made the right decision to accept the teaching job. I had learned the printing trade as a student at MSD in a shop similar to this one, but it was much more modern and much better equipped.

Rosalyn and I had been offered teaching positions at NSD when we were seniors at Gallaudet. Rosalyn was offered the position as the school's new art teacher and the girls' physical education instructor. Before our first year ended, she formed the girls' volleyball team and was their coach. I was hired as the graphic arts instructor and football and basketball coach. We had mar-

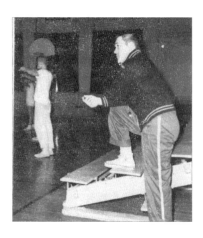

As a basketball coach at NSD, 1959.

ried that summer right after graduating from college, and spent the summer working in North Carolina. We arrived in Omaha in August, excited about our new jobs, and wasted no time coming to visit the NSD campus, where we would begin our professional lives. Fresh out of college, we were young and eager to set the world on fire. We were also a bit naive and thought we knew all the answers. It would be on this campus, over the next couple of years, where, with the guidance of some wonderful, wise, and seasoned teachers and patient school administrators, we would learn how very little we actually knew.

I opened the door, stepped into the shop, and walked slowly about the room, carefully examining each piece of equipment. Along the rear wall sat an early-nineteenth-century Intertype and a Linotype. They were those fantastic typesetting machines with over 3,000 moving parts that cast hot metal into lines of

Rosalyn as a volleyball coach at NSD, 1960.

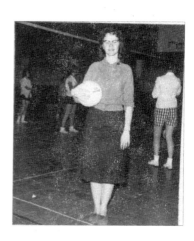

type (hence the name Linotype). These were the machines that had given thousands and thousands of deaf printers well-paying jobs in the newspaper and printing industry. The two typesetting machines I looked at were badly in need of repair. I noticed the Linotype pot, where the hot metal was heated, leaked badly, causing a buildup on one of the machine's mainsprings.

Most state schools for the deaf were pioneers in vocational training, and printing had always been a popular and well-paying trade for deaf persons. Those schools began offering training in such trades as baking, woodworking, cabinetmaking, printing, shoe repair, home economics, tailoring and dry-cleaning, barbering, painting, art, and other trades long before public schools. These programs enabled deaf graduates to learn valuable skills and move directly into the world of work. Some of the graduates eventually started their own businesses. I reflected on these things as I walked about the room where I had to somehow teach. There were hand-set type forms, tied with string borders, sitting in galleys everywhere in the shop. They were saved so it would not be necessary to hand-set them again, which was a slow and very time-consuming process. I thought it strange that with the Linotype and Intertype machines, there were so many hand-set type forms. I soon learned that the typesetting machines were in such bad condition that printing forms had to be hand-set. This was largely due to a stingy state budget.

Up to that point, the school had been under the administration of the State Board of Control, which also administered the state's prison system. The school's printshop had, in effect, been a state printshop. Rather than being a real classroom, it handled the printing needs of eighteen state institutions. This saved the state considerable money, but made teaching the students a printing trade impossible or secondary, and served little or no direct benefit to the school. In return, the state did not provide much funding to maintain or replace the shop's aging, outdated equipment. While this provided hands-on training for the students, the demand for production had become so acute that my predecessor had ended up doing most of the jobs himself because he had little or no time to teach the students. Often all but a few of the older students would sit at the long printers' tables doing their homework or talking while the instructor and a few older students rushed about the shop meeting printing deadlines.

Just the year before, the school had been placed under the direction of the State Department of Education, and printing for the state was stopped. When I was hired, I was told my job was to teach printing. As vocational teachers, it was our responsibility to teach our students not only marketable skills, but also good work habits, such as the importance of being on time, work responsibility, employer loyalty, and how to get along with co-workers. I needed to instill in each a positive outlook on life, a strong "can-do" spirit, and the value of a sense of humor. We also had to teach them how to deal with a world that was insensitive to the communication needs of deaf people. That called for a lot of patience.

I thought about my young charges and the responsibility I had to each of these young boys. I knew that many of the boys would not make it to college. Some of them would attend post-secondary vocational training programs to acquire additional training or to study a trade not offered at NSD. Many would go directly into the world of work. There they would compete with a growing number of unskilled and semiskilled workers in a shrinking labor market as technology advanced. Regardless of how well trained they were, their deafness or lack of understand-able speech would almost always be a strike against them in job competition, and often used as an excuse to deny them upward mobility during their work life.

I thought about all of this as I wandered back to the door. There I stopped and paused again as I scanned the room one last time. Suddenly, the enormity of all the responsibilities I had just inherited as a teacher hit me. I realized at that moment that what I taught my students—or didn't teach them—would have a direct impact on their lives. The knowledge I imparted, the attitudes and the work ethics I helped develop, the amount of responsibility I taught them to shoulder, to a large measure, would determine their futures. I suspect that was where my gray hair got an early start. I must have aged a couple of years during those few minutes I stood in the doorway. The excitement and challenge of working with young folks began to filter through the enormity of the task at hand and lightened the weight of responsibility. I began to realize how much all my teachers at the Missouri School had meant to me. As I thought about all this, a line from one of Alexander Pope's poems came back to me, and I began to better understand and appreciate its meaning: *"'Tis education forms the common mind: Just as the twig is bent, the trees inclin'd."*

"ORNATING" A HELPFUL NEIGHBOR

It was August 1959, when Rosalyn, my new bride, and I moved to Omaha to begin our new jobs as teachers at NSD. We had come to Omaha in August, before school opened, to get settled. Earlier that summer, with the help of Rosalyn's parents, we ordered a new mobile home from a factory in Kansas. We needed time to find a place to park it and set it up, and we wanted to be present when it arrived. We were also eager to get acquainted with the teachers and staff at the school and meet members of the local Deaf community. But the mobile home was delayed at the factory, and we were left homeless.

Fortunately for us, upon arrival, a college classmate introduced us to George and Elly Propp, who came to our rescue. Elly's Deaf parents were out of state on vacation, and she graciously suggested that we stay at her parents' home until they returned or our mobile home arrived. The house was a beautiful, two-story, well-kept old clapboard house dating back to the turn of the century. It stood on a corner lot in an older neighborhood of the city. Chairs sat on the front porch that overlooked the street and nearby intersection.

One day we experienced one of the worst thunderstorms to hit Omaha in years. Having nothing better to do, Rosalyn and I sat on the front porch and watched the downpour. The rain came down in torrents and all the water flowed down the streets to the intersection. The intersection began to flood because the water was rising faster than the sewer openings could take it. Soon the water in the intersection pooled to about two feet deep and had become impassable for cars. Grass clippings, tree branches, and street debris placed along the curbs for pickup were swept down the streets and clogged the grate openings. The more it rained, the higher the water rose.

The situation called for action. After some hesitancy, but with Rosalyn's encouragement, I removed my shoes and socks. Wearing old trousers, I waded precariously and gallantly, if not a bit foolishly, into the swirling water and drenching rain toward one of the blocked sewer outlets. I began yanking away the branches and debris and tossing them over my shoulder out of the way. I worked diligently, and with each load I discarded, the more that opening widened and the more water poured into the sewer mouth. After a while, I had managed to check the flooding.

I was about finished when I looked in the direction of the porch, where Rosalyn stood watching. Expecting some kind of commendation for my good deed, I saw her waving her arms flailing her arms instead, to get my attention. She looked alarmed and pointed her finger behind my back. Puzzled by her look of horror, I turned and glanced behind me.

There stood a stranger, plastered with twigs, clippings, and pieces of trash. He resembled a lavishly decorated Christmas tree except that he was not quite as attractive nor as green. I looked at him in embarrassment. We nodded in an awkward greeting and exchanged embarrassed smiles.

The stranger was a neighbor, Rosalyn explained later, and when he saw me attack the cause of the flood, he waded out into the intersection to give me a hand. Unfortunately, he had approached me from my blind side, not knowing I was deaf. As he got near me, I tossed an armful of litter over my shoulder, hitting him with the trash. At that point, he probably said something like, "Hey, here let me give you a hand," but, of course, I did not hear him. Meanwhile, busy as I was, I tossed another load over my shoulder. It hit him by surprise again. So he did the next logical thing; he moved to the other side behind me. Unfortunately for him, I also changed the direction of my pitch and hit him with another load. *Plop!* Another load.

At that point, I am sure he yelled, "Hey! Hey! Let me give you a hand!" as he wiped the mess from his face. But, as this situation clearly demonstrates, when words fall on deaf ears, they are never very effective. Had he thought of tapping me on the shoulder to get my attention, he would have avoided the mess. *Plop!* Another load.

It was about then that I looked toward the house and saw Rosalyn flapping her arms and turned to the Christmas tree-man behind me. Grass clippings shrouded his head and mingled in his hair. Small branches dangled from his shoulders and wet paper trash clung to his shirt.

I stood there, looking at him transfixed. I smiled weakly when I realized what had happened.

He apparently felt awkward, too. He had come out to help . . . and looked back at me with a weak smile.

"Hi," I said.

"Hi," he said.

I apologized for what had happened, pointed toward my ear, and explained that I was deaf and was not aware of his approach. He nodded his head. That much was already obvious. As he was shouting at me and trying to dodge tosses, it had dawned on him a bit too late that, like his neighbors, I, too, could not hear.

THE MAGIC OF SEPTEMBER

School finally opened in September. Opening day, when all the students returned, gradually became my favorite day of the whole school year. No matter what the year, no matter what the day, this day was always the same, yet different. Rosalyn and I enjoyed joining the students, teachers, and houseparents as we gathered in the school auditorium to witness this annual September spectacle.

We watched as the students blew into the room like a gust of prairie wind. They arrived brimming with energy, refreshed from a well-deserved break, and happy to be back among their friends. They always returned to school dressed in their new school outfits—shirts and trousers or dresses, and shoes, sneakers, or cowboy boots. They came bright-eyed, anxious, and excited with fresh-scrubbed faces and summer tans.

As the years rolled by I noticed, too, how similar this annual event was. No matter who the individuals were, the routine, the behavior, and the reactions were the same. The small children with chubby bodies the year before now stretched out into long, thin string beans and the previous skinny, long-limbed bodies filled out into handsome or pretty teenagers. Some of the kids returned a foot taller, some were heavier, and then there were those few who never seemed to grow a fraction of an inch until one school-opening day it appeared they shot up overnight. Among the older boys, there were broader shoulders, longer feet, and sprouting mustaches and, among the girls, we witnessed their magic transformation into beautiful and charming young ladies. With few exceptions, the years were kind to the children. Among the smaller kids, some front teeth were missing, and those who had left school toothless now had new teeth. New eyeglasses, dental braces, permanents, and fresh haircuts added to the changes.

School opening day also marked another milestone in our professional lives as teachers and houseparents. Among my colleagues, I noticed belt notches let farther out, and the height of high heels had shrunk. There was more gray hair—or less of it—among us and more eyeglasses, including bifocals or trifocals. Some of us moved about a tad slower than we did the year before.

Not one opening day began without some sporadic outbursts by some youngsters with unspent, uncontrollable summer energy. It always erupted when a handful of rowdy youngsters ran into the room, chasing each other. In the process, they pushed other students out of their way and knocked over folding chairs. They would be collared, reprimanded, and reminded that summer was over, and they were now back in school. For the students, such incidents were their signal that a carefree summer was finally over, and it was now back to the business of learning.

Each fall brought in a fresh crop of students with new names to be learned. I could spot the newcomers easily. They had that special "green look" only found among new students—an expression of doubt, anxiety, and uncertainty. We knew that as the year wore on and the "newness" faded with friends and acquaintances made, and routines established, the newcomers would gain confidence and begin to fit into the busy, happy environment shared with their schoolmates.

The influx of new students always brought back thoughts of the previous year's seniors. It was impossible not to think of them. We would remember the previous spring's blossoms and leaves on campus. As the school year neared the end, once again, the teachers and houseparents would find ourselves sitting in the auditorium, watching another class graduate. That moment was always bittersweet. We would watch the senior boys, with their long, lanky strides or short, heavy shuffles, and the more graceful girls as they moved across the stage, one by one, to accept their hard-earned diplomas. After receiving them and the congratulations of the superintendent and/or state official, each would then stop before descending the stage steps, look at the audience, and move the tassel to the other side of the mortar board to officially proclaim to the world—just in case there was any doubt—that they had made it. Then, a happy, million-dollar smile would flash across each face as they joyfully scampered down the steps into a new world. Some would throw their beaming parents, friends, and relatives a kiss or an I-LOVE-YOU sign. After the ceremony, the seniors marched out of the auditorium and stood in line to receive congratulations from everyone before departing from the campus one last time. And, when they left, a little bit of our lives went with them.

There were always those students in whom you had the utmost confidence and the highest expectations to succeed. At times some of them would disappoint us and fall short of our expectations while others whom we had doubted about would beat the odds and excel beyond our wildest expectations. The persistent "whys?" we always badgered ourselves with were part of the puzzle of the teaching profession.

At long last, the September procession into the auditorium ended, all the greetings, hellos, and hand waves had been exchanged, and the lively mass of excited human energy finally subdued. The superintendent then arose with as much dignity as he could muster and walked to the podium at the center of the stage to announce the beginning of the new school year and to extend an official warm welcome to everyone. He shared information about summer activities and the school's status in the coming year then returned to his seat. Next, the principal followed—he extended greetings and introduced the new teachers and houseparents. Then he got down to the business of assigning all the students to their classes. Happy, excited faces began to turn into tense expressions as class placement was called and, one by one, the students gathered with their classmates and new teachers and departed.

Surely, this is an annual event that takes place in schools throughout America on a particular fall day. But there was one slight difference at schools like ours. The day before, the students had packed their suitcases, left their homes and families, and come to live at NSD because our school, like many other schools for deaf children, was a state residential school. Rosalyn and I often reflected on our own experiences of leaving home to attend such a school. We remembered the moments of parting from our families and smiled knowingly at how quickly that tearful moment was swept away by the excitement of a new school year. The family parting was always a more heart-wrenching experience for the parents than for the children. After the sadness of the moment had passed, the students quickly adapted to their new environment and routine.

As teachers, we also looked forward to the new year and our responsibilities with excitement and anticipation. We learned how we shaped the lives of our young charges and, in turn, were shaped by them. Our lives were touched by each youngster we worked with and became intertwined in theirs. How their joys became our joys, their disappointments, our disappointments. We shared their secrets, doubts, and dreams. We were with them in triumphs and defeats.

Being witness to this annual September spectacle on school opening day, year in and year out, was one of the rewards of being a teacher. It was a special privilege to have a box seat in this grandstand of life and to witness the transformations of these young people as, one by one, class after class, they climbed up the learning ladder on their journey into tomorrow. Many of us felt we could not have picked a more rewarding profession.

JILL "HI-J-A-C-K-S" ME

I was returning from the school mailroom and headed down the hallway to the printshop in the vocational building when seven-year-old Jill ran out of her classroom to greet me with her teacher Mrs. Brasel in hot pursuit.

HI, J-A-C-K! Jill signed and fingerspelled to me proudly, a small smirk on her narrow face.

HI! I responded, smiling, signing in a large circular motion with my hand to give her an extra big greeting.

Mrs. Brasel, who had just caught up with Jill, saw what had transpired, and looked on in dismay. Her lower jaw had dropped and a startled look covered her face. She put her hands on her hips, then with a stern look at Jill, scolded: "Why, Jill! That's not right!"

Amused, I stood silently and watched the exchange, trying hard to suppress a laugh.

WHHHHYYYY? signed Jill in a long, slow, exaggerated manner. She shook her head sideways in embarrassment as if caught saying a bad word. "Why?" she asked again, "That *is* his name!"

"Because," responded Mrs. Brasel, every bit the teacher, "you do not call an adult by his *first* name." She paused, then curiosity overcoming her, asked, "Where did you learn his first name?"

"I saw it in the *Tiger*," signed Jill. The *Tiger* was our school yearbook and had all the students' and teachers' pictures and names. "I know your husband's first name, too," she added in an attempt to get off the hook with a little flattery. "It's D-E-W-E-Y!"

Mrs. Brasel's mouth flew open again. But Jill's attempt didn't work. This time Mrs. Brasel clenched her fists and put them on her hips, then shook her index finger at Jill, "Jill! That's not polite. You don't call the principal by his first name, either!"

I was enjoying the banter.

"Why?" asked Jill, trying to look as naive and innocent as she could. She kicked the toe of one shoe on the floor as the embarrassed look returned to her face.

"Because you are supposed to use Mr. or Miss or Mrs. and their last names when you greet or talk to older persons," Mrs. Brasel signed as she spoke. "You cannot—it is not polite—to use an older person's first name. Do you understand?"

Reluctantly, Jill slowly nodded her head that she did. O-H . . . O-K, she fingerspelled, a look of disappointment. She turned, looked at me, smiled again, and said, HI, M-R. G-A-N-N-O-N.

The bell rang, and the lights flashed to signal recess. Mrs. Brasel and I watched as Jill turned around and skipped down the hallway on her way outside to play. As she went out the door, in strode sixteen-year-old Ken Eurek, the school's star quarterback and one of Jill's idols. Ken held the door open for Jill.

As Jill exited, she turned and looked up at Ken, then glanced in our direction and with a devilish look on her face, she bowed curtly and signed and fingerspelled to Ken, THANK YOU, M-R. E-U-R-E-K. Ken watched her leave, then turned and looked around to be sure he was the one she had just spoken to. Seeing no one else, he shrugged his shoulders and walked down the hall, no doubt wondering why things had suddenly become so formal at the school.

MISS TRUKKEN AND HER "HEARING" GLASSES

Miss Trukken taught second grade in the primary unit. She was the most considerate teacher in the whole school. Not a birthday, wedding anniversary, or illness passed without a card or thoughtful gesture from her.

Miss Trukken was an orphan. I do not know what happened to her parents, but it was obvious to all of us that she considered NSD her "real" family, and she treated everyone with love and affection. She was jumpy, excitable, happy, and very expressive. She didn't walk across a room; rather, she bounced. She was also very hard of hearing. She was one of those persons who had progressive deafness and, although she had been a teacher of deaf children for many years, she found it difficult to come to terms with her *own* hearing loss.

The denial of hearing loss is not at all unique among older persons, but for a teacher of deaf and hard of hearing children, one would think she would have responded differently. As she advanced in years, her hearing loss became noticeably worse.

Many of us realized she was not only embarrassed about it but having difficulty admitting she needed help.

To make matters worse, while Miss Trukken signed fairly well, she had poor receptive skills. She had learned sign language only after coming to NSD, and she had difficulty reading and understanding most signers. Often she nodded to indicate that she understood what was being signed when in truth, she didn't.

In a sense, people with severe hearing loss and little or no sign language skills lived in a no man's land caught somewhere between the deaf and hearing worlds, being a member of both yet finding it most difficult to fit into either. These individuals lack sufficient hearing to keep up with spoken speech and they do not possess adequate sign language receptive skills to follow a signed conversation. As a result, they often get lost in a conversation, easily become bored, and sometimes fall asleep during a signed or spoken conversation, something Miss Trukken often did.

When those tiny new hearing aids with the auditory mechanisms built into eyeglass frames appeared on the market, Miss Trukken was among the first to buy a pair. They were perfect for her because she could conceal the receiver with her hairdo. While the new hearing aid was helpful, it did not completely solve her hearing loss because she was not getting all the auditory input she needed.

All this, of course, did not detract one bit from the wonderful person that she was. With her familiar spry gait, she bounced about the school building and across the campus with boundless energy and laughter in her heart, spreading joy and good cheer in her wake. She resembled a person who didn't have a care or problem in the world. And she loved to entertain. She invited her class and members of the NSD family to her home for dinners, receptions, and parties.

One evening she invited Rosalyn, me, and our good friends, Frank and Ginny, to her home for dinner. Until that evening, we had not known she had acquired a pair of those new hearing aid glasses. As most hearing aid users are aware, they are assistive devices that require time to get used to. It turned out to be the evening Miss Trukken inadvertently acknowledged to us that she had a hearing loss. Arriving at her house, we thought it a bit strange to note that she was not wearing her glasses as usual, but we did not inquire about them.

Following a sumptuous, delicious dinner, all of us sat around in a circle chatting. It soon became evident that as the signed and spoken conversation wore on, Miss Trukken was not keeping pace. She began to nod her head drowsily, fighting off sleep. The four of us noticed this and looked at each other and smiled knowingly.

Suddenly the doorbell rang. The persistent *Ring! Ring! Ring!* jarred Miss Trukken awake, and she bounced up from the sofa and sprang to the door. It was the newspaper boy. He had come to collect payment for his delivery services. He informed Miss Trukken of her bill, but not wearing her hearing aid, she did not get the amount. Ginny, who is hearing, interpreted the exchange for us.

"What?" Miss Trukken asked.

The newspaper boy explained again the purpose of his presence.

"Oh," said Miss Trukken, "How much?"

The young fellow repeated the amount of the bill.

But Miss Trukken didn't get it. "How much?" she asked again. The newspaper boy patiently repeated himself for the fourth time.

By the look on her face, we knew that Miss Trukken still did not understand what he had said. There was a long, awkward pause. The youth stood there at the door, waiting uneasily. Finally, Miss Trukken admitted, "I'm sorry—I can't hear you." She held up her index finger and said, "Please wait here and let me get my glasses."

The four of us glanced at the newspaper boy. We knew what she was referring to—her eyeglasses with the hearing aid, but the young boy didn't understand. A perplexed look crept over his face as he stood there puzzled. No doubt he was wondering, "How does a person hear with eyeglasses?!"

The boy finally got his money.

BRIAN TELLS ME ABOUT TOMORROW THREE

Tomorrow, tomorrow, tomorrow, three! Brian signed excitedly to me as he entered my classroom one morning. I did a double-take. At first, I thought I was seeing another version of William Shakespeare's *Macbeth*, but then I realized that Brian was much too young for that.

say, what? I signed to Brian.

It was just after mail call, and Brian had received a letter from home with some good news.

mother sending box tomorrow three! he exclaimed in signs. I feigned ignorance because he was not using correct English grammar as was then the school's policy.

tomorrow, three, what? I repeated, my brows furrowed to show I did not understand.

yes! Brian pumped his fist, still overjoyed. tomorrow three!

tomorrow three . . . ? understand zero, I signed to Brian, playing along.

With a heavy sigh and an impatient frown that said, "I can't believe how dumb you are," he pointed at one finger and told me to watch.

TODAY, MONDAY! he glanced at me with his eyebrows raised in that familiar questioning facial expression that most of his teachers used to ask, "Do you understand?"

I nodded.

TOMORROW TUESDAY! pointing to his second finger as he kept count, and eyeing me again with that questioning look. I nodded again.

TOMORROW, TOMORROW WEDNESDAY! he pointed to his third finger. Then he summarized what he had just told me like his teachers always did.

TODAY—ONE; TODAY, TOMORROW—TWO; TODAY, TOMOR-ROW, TOMORROW—THREE! he signed. UNDERSTAND?!

OHHH . . . I acknowledged. "Oh, I understand. That's great!"

"Yes!" Brian exclaimed satisfied that I had finally gotten the point and probably wondering what had taken me so long.

YES, TOMORROW, TOMORROW, TOMORROW THREE! he signed to the world at large, gleefully rubbing his hands together as he put on one of the long printer's aprons and went to his assign-ment. He had it all figured out. He was counting the days until that box of candy and other homemade goodies from his mother arrived.

MARTY, THE "EXPERT" SIGNER

Marty was the new vocational rehabilitation counselor assigned to work with deaf clients in Nebraska. He came to the school often to counsel our seniors, which was how the two of us became acquainted and then good friends.

Marty wasted little time taking sign language classes because he realized that to succeed in his job, he had to be able to communicate effectively with his deaf clients. He picked up signs fast and took pride in his progress. Unfortunately, he was one of those hearing persons who, after only a few classes, considered his sign skills much better than they actually were. Deaf people frequently encounter individuals like Marty. While we appreciate their interest and desire to communicate with us, it requires a good deal of patience and tolerance on our part to live with them until their day of reckoning arrives when they realize the true limitations of their sign skills.

Marty's day of reckoning arrived sooner than most of us anticipated. Thank goodness.

One day he was meeting with one of the seniors, a polite young woman. During the session, he could not suppress the temptation to show off his newly acquired sign skills. "I'm just learning sign," he signed to her, implying modesty as he moved his fingers and mouthed the words. "Please be patient with me." Then he would stop signing and inquire: "You follow me okay?"

The young deaf woman nodded her head and signed YES.

Encouraged and feeling good, Marty continued. They had met to review the results of the young lady's job skills evaluation.

Midway through the discussion, Marty paused and asked again in signs as he spoke, "You understand me okay?"

Again, the young lady signed YES as she nodded her head. Buoyed by his success, he became fired up, and the sin of over-confidence propelled him to start using all the new, unique expressions he had recently learned. As they progressed through the evaluation, the young lady nodded her head from time to time to indicate that she was following the conversation.

Marty was feeling so proud of himself. He began to visualize the young lady telling all her deaf friends how impressed she was with that "new vocational rehabilitation counselor *who signed so well*. He even knows ASL expressions!" she would tell them. Word would spread quickly, as it always did through the deaf grapevine, and who knew, he might even be asked to interpret for members of the Deaf community. He wouldn't be the least surprised if the local television station requested that he interpret the evening news and other special programs for the benefit of deaf viewers. Imagine, he thought, what the exposure to thousands and thousands of television viewers all over the state could do for his status and where that could lead. Who knew, he might even get tapped for the state vocational rehabilitation director's job when that position became vacant thanks to his fame, impressive knowledge of signs, and sensitivity to deafness. Marty smiled as these thoughts ran through his head.

When the two had completed the job evaluation, Marty concluded the discussion and asked her one more time, "Did you have any problems understanding me?"

"No, no problem at all," the young lady said.

Marty tried again for some ego strokes, "And all my signs were clear, right? Did I use any signs wrong?"

"Oh . . ." she said. Marty was puzzled. Then, shaking her head, she apologized and said, "I really don't know. I didn't notice your signs. I was lipreading you."

TED'S "PUBLIC" GIRLFRIEND

The signs for the words "public" and "hearing" are often the same. The sign is formed by rotating the index finger in front of and under the lower lip to indicate words "rolling" out of the mouth. To differentiate between the two words, the receiver relies on the context of the message or reads the sender's lips if he or she mouths the words. Sometimes these two words get mixed up. I remember the day Ted, who had just entered his teens, came into the shop following Christmas break and proudly announced that he had a new hearing girlfriend. But, in relaying the good news, he mouthed the word "public" instead of "hearing."

I repeated what he had told me. "Question, you have a new *public* girlfriend?" I signed.

"Yes!" he signed, beaming, "a *public* girlfriend." He saw my quizzical look and, mistaking that for disapproval, started defending his choice.

"What! You don't like public girls?" he asked me.

"I don't know," I replied. "I don't think I would want a *public* girlfriend myself."

"Why?" he quickly demanded. "They're better than deaf girls!"

"Really?" I signed again, playing along with him, showing by my facial expression that I was giving his question a lot of thought, but had my doubts.

The other boys in the shop noticed our discussion and gathered around to watch.

"You like deaf better?" Ted persisted.

"Doesn't matter," I signed, "but I still don't think I would want a *public* girlfriend." I emphasized "public" as I signed and mouthed it.

SICK ME YOU, Ted signed, using the popular "your teasing makes me sick" expression while looking at me confused.

"Ted," I asked, "what does public mean?"

"Same as hearing," Ted signed, pointing to his ear.

"Not always," I replied, and asked the other boys if they knew the difference. They shook their heads.

The word "hearing" was easy to explain because it was the opposite of "deaf." To explain "public," though, I needed to give some examples, so I picked the public library.

"Do you go to the public library at home?" I asked Ted and the boys. Most of them nodded.

"Why is it called a public library?" I asked.

Ted furrowed his brow. Some of the boys shrugged their shoulders to indicate they weren't sure. I explained, "It is a public library because our tax money supports it and so everyone can use it. It's free. It belongs to all of us."

Ted and some of the boys began to use the OHHH sign, showing that they were beginning to understand. I gave them other examples: public schools, public restrooms, public parks.

Ted and the boys got the picture. They had a look of disgust at how simple the meaning was.

"So, you have a public girlfriend, right?" I asked, turning my attention back to Ted.

NO . . . NO . . . NO . . . Ted signed, blushing, obviously feeling silly now that he knew the difference.

GENE INVENTS HIS OWN VERB

School policy required all students to write about the activities they had been engaged in during class at the end of each vocational shop period. This prompted vocabulary development and exercises in English usage, and helped the students remember the names of the tools they used or the machines they operated. Sometimes in writing their assignments, when a student did not know or remember a word, he would use the signed version as a substitute and try to translate it into an English word, as Gene did one morning.

Gene was fourteen years old, rather old for his class, and small for his age. Standing on tiptoe, I doubt he could have stretched to more than five feet. It appeared he had forgotten to grow. He was a cute little guy with big, dark brown eyes, a round, dimpled, happy face, and a crewcut. Despite the shortness of his hair, it still managed to grow every which way.

Gene was a jumpy, excitable little fellow, seldom without a broad smile on his face. Never could he sit or stand still. He was what at that time was called "low verbal," meaning that he had a very limited vocabulary and a weak grasp of English or written language, but he signed well. Gene was one of the many deaf children we received at NSD who had languished for years in a local public school where his deafness had either gone undetected or was ignored, causing him and students like him to lose the best learning years of their lives. Often when the parents of these children finally came to terms with their child's deafness and realized that their child was not developing as well as he or she could in the local school program, they sent their child to our school and/or they finally learned to communicate with their child using sign language. By then, many of these deaf children had passed the critical learning years of their lives; it was often too late for most of them to catch up. They would spend the rest of their lives with their true educational potential undeveloped. Gene was one such child and had come to NSD only as a teenager.

Sign is to most deaf people what speech is to hearing people. In either situation, it is easy to sign or speak a word without knowing how to spell it. That was Gene's situation. He had picked up a good grasp of sign language after his arrival and was able to communicate well with his peers, but when it came to writing, he did not know many words or how to spell them. Gene, like many other students, found it easier to identify and remember nouns—the names of concrete objects—than to remember unseen verbs.

On that particular day, the end of the class period came and went. All the other students had completed their writing assignments and left. Gene sat at the long printer's folding table alone, with a long pencil in one hand, scratching his tousled hair with the other, as he stared at the sheet of paper. I was at my desk doing paperwork and out of the corner of my eye, I watched as he fidgeted in his chair, alternately holding his chin in his hand, looking at the ceiling, and staring at his unfinished writing assignment. His work assignment for that morning had been to put away the printer's furniture—wooden blocks of different sizes that were used to lock in type forms for the plate press—and to sweep the shop. His last sentence seemed to have him stumped, but he did not want my help or he would have come over, tapped me on the shoulder, and asked. Clearly, he wanted to handle it himself, and I saw no reason to interfere. He sat struggling and squirming as the long hand on the wall clock crept closer and closer to the time for his next class.

Suddenly, as if a light had been turned on, he sat upright, his face brightened in triumph. He scribbled something on the paper, hastily slid off the chair, placed his essay in the assignment box, caught my attention with a cheery goodbye wave, and scooted out the door.

Curious, I went over to the assignment box, sifted through all the papers, and pulled out Gene's. I soon found the word he had been struggling with. He didn't know the word for "swept." I smiled at his creativity as I looked out the window and watched him return to the school building in his familiar hop-skip-walk. He had written: "I *broomed* the floor."

"FORGET IT!"

Thomas Scott Cuscaden Sr. was a big, burly man. He stood over six feet tall and weighed more than 250 pounds. He was born deaf and lost the sight in one eye due to high fever. His name sign was "F-on-the-chest." Where he got the "F" no one knows. Scott's mother, Dr. Gertrude Cuscaden, was one of the first female doctors in Omaha.

As a student, Scott had excelled in sports. He was an all-around athlete and had helped start the football and basketball teams at NSD while starring on them, and was also a regular on the baseball team. In college, he was the leading tackle and captain of the Gallaudet football team and was twice selected to the Southeast Atlantic Coast All-Star Football Team. During World War I, Scott, like many other deaf persons, worked for Goodyear in Ohio. He captained the well-known "Goodyear Silents," the semiprofessional football team composed of deaf athletes who were also employed by the rubber plants in Akron during the war years. The team racked up a record of sixty-five victories, six defeats, and three ties, and in 1917 won the Central Ohio Championship. Scott was the first Nebraskan to be inducted into the American Athletic Association of the Deaf Hall of Fame.

Scott's wife, Nellie, was a beautiful, gentle woman who was also a patient, dedicated teacher. Her name sign was similar to her husband's, except hers was "N-on-the-chest." She had been deafened by scarlet fever when she was seven years old. Like Scott, she was a graduate of NSD and had attended Gallaudet, but was forced to leave after only one year when her father died. She had a special talent for reaching children who came to NSD late from public school programs and were far behind academically or who had learning disabilities. Nellie had a way of winning these students' confidence and helping them achieve as much as possible during their brief stay at the school. Nellie's students knew they could always count on her in time of need, and many of them returned to visit her long after they had left school.

Scott and Nellie had four children—three deaf and one hearing. All three deaf children were graduates of NSD and Gallaudet University. Both Scott and Nellie were retired when Rosalyn and I first met them. We had stayed at their house while they were away during our first week in Omaha, where I had "ornated" that neighbor.

Scott wrote the alumni news column that appeared regularly in the *Nebraska Journal*, which the boys printed. He stopped by the shop each month to drop off his column and to remind me, quoting lyrics from an old song as he was fond of doing, that "everybody works, but Father." It was during these visits that we became good friends. On one occasion, he told me the following story.

In 1945, Scott was hired as the dean of boys at the nearby Iowa School for the Deaf (ISD) in Council Bluffs, a position he held for thirteen years until his retirement. One fall day after ISD opened, a petite woman with a tall, reluctant young son in tow came into his office in the boys' dormitory. She burst into the office and immediately began talking. Scott, who had attended NSD when it was required by law—the only such law in the nation—to teach all deaf children by the oral method, had no usable speech. He got up from his desk, walked around it, and extended his hand in greeting. Towering over the woman, he looked down at her. When she persisted in talking excitedly and rapidly, he courteously informed her that he was deaf by pointing an index finger to one ear and shaking his head.

The mother looked up at him, startled, and heaved a sigh. "Oh!" she said, placing a hand on her chest, a sympathetic and disappointed, helpless look on her face. Her son stood behind her, leaning against the door frame, bored, his gaze wandering about the room. Scott picked up a pad of paper from his desk and pulled out a pen from his shirt pocket and handed them to her. She nodded her head appreciatively, took them, and began to write furiously.

"This is my son, Rodney . . ." she began and went on to explain at length how her son had been taught in an oral day school by the "oral approach," which the family preferred, and now that she was transferring him to ISD, she wanted to make it clear that she didn't want him to learn sign language. To emphasize how strongly she felt about the matter, she drew three lines under the words "not," "learn," and "signs" and ended the sentence with three exclamation points.

As the mother wrote, Scott looked over her shoulders at Rodney and studied him. Scott extended warm greetings, welcomed him to the dormitory, and asked him about himself. Except for a glance and a grudging nod, there was no other response from the boy. He looked quickly about the room, purposely avoiding Scott's attention. Scott immediately sensed the problem. Here was another orally taught and communication-deprived deaf child. Scott began to seethe with anger.

Finally, the mother finished writing and handed the note to Scott and stared up at him as he read it. "No signs!" she repeated orally, shaking her index finger in a scolding manner at Scott. She pointed the same finger toward her lips, "Talk! Talk!" she said, nodding her head aggressively.

Scott looked at the mother then at her son and nodded slowly and sadly, indicating he understood her request. He could see little or no communication between mother and son, and the mother was still insisting on imposing a communication barrier. Instead of getting to know her son and understanding his needs as a deaf person, she had unknowingly become part of his problems with her adamant, restrictive insistence on one form of communication and depriving him of free access to information. It contributed to his frustration, his withdrawal from family participation, and he developed a tendency to dwell in his own private world and respond only when spoken to. Scott immediately sensed a lack of social skills and a crippling inability to express himself.

Scott nodded again. He had encountered this situation many times before but could do little about it. In the past, he had argued with these naive parents so often that the school superintendent had called him into his office, reprimanded him, and told him to stop. Scott knew that the only way to restrain his anger was to say nothing. He nodded that he understood what she had said but did not respond.

Getting no other reply, the mother kissed the boy on the cheek, waved her index finger at him, told him to be good, and bade him a hasty goodbye. Rodney watched his mother go, his face blank, then turned his attention to notices on the bulletin board.

Scott picked up Rodney's suitcase, tapped him on the shoulder, and gestured for him to follow. Scott led him upstairs to the intermediate boys' floor, showed him his bedroom, and then took the shy, withdrawn boy to the lobby area called the "reading room." There Scott blinked the room lights to get the other boys' attention, introduced the newcomer, and returned to his office.

In the ensuing weeks, Scott made no effort to restrict Rodney from learning sign language. He knew from experience that that was impossible because sign language is the natural language of deaf people. Scott watched as the boy began to pick up signs and express himself. The lad became more expressive, outgoing, more involved, and more interested in the world around him. As his communication skills improved, he started flooding Scott and the other houseparents with questions. He made friends and began to blend into the group. As the months passed, Scott could hardly believe the transformation he saw take place in Rodney, who was gradually changing from a disinterested, solemn, withdrawn youth into a happy participant in the activities around him.

The changes in Rodney were so natural that Scott thought nothing further about them until that day in January when all the students returned following the winter break. By chance,

Scott glanced down the long dormitory hallway and saw Rodney's mother striding in his direction. Rodney walked cheerfully alongside her, greeting his friends in sign language as he went. "What a different kid from the one who had arrived earlier that fall," Scott thought, but seeing the determined walk and the frown on Rodney's mother's face, he sensed a confrontation coming. He ducked into his office, where he pretended to concentrate on paperwork. He was hoping she would see he was busy and go talk with another houseparent, but that ploy didn't work.

She flew into his office like a whirlwind. She plunked her big black purse on Scott's desk, capturing his attention, nodded her head in a curt greeting, held up her index finger signaling for Scott to wait a minute, and dug through her purse. Finally, she found what she was looking for—a pad and pencil. She took them out and began writing furiously.

Rodney, meanwhile, waved at Scott upon entering the office, walked over and gave him a bear hug, and excitedly started telling Scott what he did over the holidays, all in sign language. Scott cringed and quickly moved between Rodney and his mother and signed for Rodney to calm down, hoping that his mother, who was still busy writing, would not notice all the signing. But Rodney, too excited and with too much to talk about, just kept rambling on. The mother finished writing and handed the pad to Scott. On it she had written, "Remember when I came here last fall, and I told you I did not want my son learning sign language?"

Scott slowly nodded his head. Of course, he remembered. How could he forget! The mother snatched the pad out of his hands and started writing again. "Uh-oh," Scott thought to himself, here comes trouble. But, the mother only wrote for a short time, handed the pad back to Scott, and fixed her eyes on him as he read the pad. She had written only two words and, once again, she had underlined them and ended her comments with three exclamation points.

"Forget it!!!" she had written.

After finishing the story, Scott left the shop, and I returned to reading some galley proofs. Momentarily, the shop lights blinked, and I looked up and saw Scott back in the doorway, his hands on the light switches to get my attention. When he saw I was looking at him, he signed to me across the room: "By the way, Rodney is now a houseparent at a school for the deaf." He turned around not waiting for a response, waved his hand over his head in a farewell motion, as deaf people sometimes do, and walked out the door.

THE BOYS OF SEPTEMBER, OCTOBER, AND NOVEMBER

Following the previous dismal season, Coach Bryant and I inherited a new crop of ambitious youngsters, and our football fortunes took an upswing.

Eddie played guard. He was short, round, and fat with the olive complexion of his Italian ancestors. Eddie was a good-natured lad, and the team loved to tease him. He always had a big smile, and no matter how hard he tried, he could never really get mad with anyone. He would pout a few seconds to tell the others he was "upset," then, unable to hold his look, break out in a smile. We gave him the name sign PIZZA because that was his favorite food.

Alan was tall and slim and had very long legs. When he ran, all you could see were those long legs cartwheeling down the field. He played end, and, although he was an average receiver, he was outstanding on defense. He was one of the boys on the team who went on to college. Alan's mother, one of our best fans, attended most of our games. She was also an excellent bread baker. During a fundraiser, she donated some of her homemade bread for the senior class's cakewalk. I had given a ticket to a student who didn't have one, and she promptly won the loaf of bread I wanted. When Alan's mother heard what had happened, she baked another loaf and sent it to me at school.

Pat was a very poor academic achiever, caused by a late-in-life transfer to our school as a teenager. He could neither read nor write and had woeful communication skills. His parents and the public school officials in his hometown said they didn't know there was a school for deaf children in the state. As a consequence, Pat spent the rest of his life paying for that ignorance.

Except for his weight, Pat was ideal fullback material. He was lean and fast and tough as nails, but he had difficulty understanding and remembering the offensive plays. He was also just learning to communicate in sign language. The quarterback

Rosalyn as an art teacher.

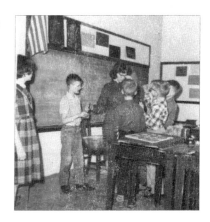

would call a play, and Pat would either not understand it or not remember what the play involved, go the wrong way, and foul up everything. I tried anything I could think of to help him understand the system and remember the plays, all to no avail. I even tried writing the plays and taping them to his wrist so he could glance at them as reminders, but that didn't work either, so I switched him to defense. There he excelled. He became what I called our expert "shoestring" tackler. If you can visualize a tall tree crashing to the ground after being cut, you can picture how ball carriers hit the sod when Pat tackled them.

Terry and Bob were halfbacks. Both weighed about the same, but Terry was the shorter of the two. They were tough, fast, good ball carriers and receivers. They made it possible for us to diversify our attack, and made critical yardage when we found ourselves in bad third-down situations. They also caught short passes and drew the defense away from Doug, our star receiver, when the other team started to gang up on him.

Despite his small size, Doug was an amazing athlete. He was the best receiver I had ever seen on a high school team. He had excellent hands, good speed, and a very flexible running form. His hands seemed to attract footballs like magnets attract metal. After witnessing some of his "impossible" catches, I could have sworn he had a ball magnet in his hands! He could jump between two taller defenders on the run and snatch the ball out of their grasp. He also made unbelievable diving saves, catching the ball inches from the ground. In addition to all this, he and his younger deaf brother and sister were quiet, modest, and unassuming, but they all were terrific athletes.

Cliff was a big, heavyset farm boy. His feet pointed slightly outward from each other, and he walked with a waddle and sometimes made the school's old wooden floor vibrate. When Cliff first joined the team, he had great difficulty controlling his emotions. If he became frustrated, he would burst into tears or lose his temper. When he became angry or upset, he would yank off his helmet, slam it on the ground, and stomp off the field in a huff. As he grew older, however, he matured, mastered his emotions, and developed confidence in himself and his capabilities. He became an excellent lineman and a fine young man.

Ken was a coach's dream. He was an outstanding all-around athlete from a religious, hard-working farm family. He was tall, strong, dark, and handsome, and had a beautiful, broad smile and dimples. He was a smart lad, game savvy, a fierce competitor, cool under pressure, and an excellent, unassuming leader. He was another member of the team who went on to college, and he became a coach at a school for the deaf.

For a star, Ken was unusually modest and a perfect model for the younger children who idolized him. Being a star, however, had its drawbacks as Ken was to learn. One day he approached me in the printshop and lamented, "I don't like being a star!" Surprised by the comment, I asked why.

"Because all the children are always after me and always watching everything I do. I can't be myself!" he lamented.

I chuckled. "Tough luck," I signed. "That's the price of glory!"

Ken, Doug, Bob, and Terry were classmates. When they were in grade school, I used to watch them outside the printshop windows as they gathered with the other boys on the playground to play football during recess, during lunch hour, and after school. I watched them grow up and develop their skills, camaraderie, team spirit, and competitiveness. These boys were just some of the many fine young folks I had the privilege to get to know and work with. Working with students like these was one of the "fringe benefits" of being a teacher and a coach. There were, of course, many others.

Ken, Doug, Bob, and Terry had another classmate, who also loved sports, but was unable to play. He had a far greater impact on our football team's success than he would ever realize. And, his name was Gary.

YOUNG GARY'S COURAGE AND MAGIC

Although it happened many years ago, I still remember the shock I felt the day I grasped Gary's arm. It felt as if I were holding on to a broomstick. In addition to being deaf, Gary had muscular dystrophy, a deadly disease that eats away at the body's muscles. Gary was twelve years old when he enrolled in my graphic arts class. He was little more than skin and bones. He was tall for his age and so thin, with high protruding cheekbones, heavy eyebrows, and a thick shock of dark hair. His back curved in the shape of an "s"—his hips pointed in one direction and his shoulders in another. He walked very slowly and very carefully to keep from falling. When he fell, and he often did, he would just fold up and collapse on the floor, looking like a pile of rags. It was a heartrending and sickening sight. The boys and I would rush to Gary to help him up, but he would slowly raise one arm and, with his hand, adamantly wave us away. Then, with a set jaw and a determined look on his face, he would slowly unfold his crumpled body, get on his hands and knees, crawl to the nearest table or piece of furniture, and climb to his feet while we looked on.

Because of Gary's inability to control his balance, I was deathly afraid of permitting him near any operating machines. I had nightmares of seeing him lose his balance and accidentally fall into one of the presses. To reduce the chances of such an accident, I offered him the opportunity to work in the new darkroom, where I taught him to develop film and make prints. He could lean against and hold on to a long, sturdy stainless steel sink while he worked. When he got tired, he could sit on the high stool we had added. He was not only learning a skill but also contributing to the class. I could see that he enjoyed the work, and it gave him prestige and an important sense of responsibility that he took very seriously. Often he came to class and went straight to the darkroom, and I had to double-check to be sure he had arrived. I always found him busy at work. He became a fairly good darkroom technician. That's where I learned that pride was good medicine.

Gary, of course, couldn't play sports, but unknown to him and others, he made a real contribution to the success of our football team. One Monday afternoon, after a weekend loss, the football team was going through a listless practice on Booth Field. Booth Field, named for an early NSD superintendent, was located at the bottom of a long, steep incline, past the school's power plant and the old orchard. We had to watch our step going down the rock-strewn hill, and it was a long hard climb back up, especially after a tough workout.

That afternoon, the players were demoralized. Nothing we did seemed to go right. The desire, the spark, and the motivation were all missing. Bryant, the other coach, and I weren't feeling very up ourselves when a movement on the hill caught our attention. One by one, we looked to see in the distance a familiar figure coming slowly down the hill. It was Gary. I could recognize his teetering gait a mile away! He lifted one leg, and since he had little or no muscle control, the front of his foot immediately dropped forward with his toes pointing to the ground. Then, swaying precariously, he carefully set that foot down a few inches in front of him, lifted the other leg, and repeated the process with his other foot. That way he slowly and cautiously walked and made the trip down the hill. It was a very dangerous trip for him because, if he fell, he could get hurt, and there were not many things he could grab ahold of to pull himself back up.

Soon the whole team's gaze was on the hillside. It took a tough stomach to watch, yet we all stood there, our eyes transfixed on Gary. We looked on in silence, both with anxiety and admiration. Despite the risk involved and effort it took him to make the trek to the football field and the even harder climb back up, Gary came down as often as he could to stand on the sidelines to watch his school and classmates practice, doing what he could never do.

He didn't realize it, but on this particular afternoon, he jarred the team out of its exhaustion and instilled in it a renewed spirit. Bryant and I immediately sensed a change when we turned our attention back to practice. As if we were a single body, suddenly all of us realized how fortunate we all were to be able to play football. Most of us had always taken our strong arms and legs for granted. Now we realized how fortunate we were to be able to run and block and tackle, to fall and jump right back up, ready for more of the same, something Gary would never do even once. It was as if Gary had waved a magic wand over us and created a sudden, amazing transformation of the lethargic team we were only moments ago. The boys' spirit and determination returned, they began to hustle, and the plays began to click.

The rest of the afternoon passed quickly, and, in the weeks that followed, the team began to win one game after another. We ended that season with six victories and only two losses, one of the best records in the school's history. We had no way of knowing it then, of course, but greater things lay in store for us. And I credit much of that success to Gary's contribution to his team. That was Gary's magic.

I have thought of Gary many times since I left NSD. He was neither an athlete nor an outstanding student, yet he was a star in his own remarkable way. He simply fought to live. None of the young people I have ever worked with stand out more for sheer courage and guts than Gary.

On my return to the school some years ago, I inquired about Gary and was told that his body continued to deteriorate so badly he began to use a wheelchair. To make matters worse, NSD was then inaccessible to wheelchairs, so he had to leave. That, I know, was a devastating blow to him. He became bedridden just before he died.

On learning the news of his passing, I turned away with a heavy heart and misty eyes. Our spunky little fighter had lost his battle with muscular dystrophy, but in the process, he had won another. He had captured the hearts of all of us who had had the privilege to know him. I would remember him and his courage always.

FOUR-SEVEN MAKES THE TEAM

We had only nine players on our eight-man football team one year, but what a season! It was a coach's worst nightmare, and a season any coach would want the most to forget. We lost all five of our games and were outscored 298 to 59 points. Our opponents buried us by such lopsided scores as 85–20 and 56–6. Yet, amazingly, light pierced all that gloom. That was because Denny—or FOUR-SEVEN (his height and his name sign)—made the team. Without FOUR-SEVEN, there would have been no football season that year at NSD where I coached with Rick, my assistant coach.

All our young players, including FOUR-SEVEN, showed us their determination, their stubbornness, and their refusal to give up. They gave their all despite moments of frustration, and hung on to the bitter end of every single game. Their refusal to quit when the odds were overwhelming and the score was outrageous earned them respect and admiration. They taught the coaches and the fans alike a simple lesson in courage. It was to their credit that we did not cancel a single game.

FOUR-SEVEN, in particular, stood out during this weary season. To call Denny a player was really stretching things a bit. He was old enough to play to be sure, and he packed enough fight and energy to make any team, but he was physically a mite too small to make an average football team. We had the option of including him on the team or canceling the whole season. All the boys, including Denny, wanted to play—and playing with only one substitute was allowed during those days—so we played.

Denny was a freshman that year. He was a perfect reflection of that season's Tiger spirit. As the only substitute on the team, when he wasn't prancing excitedly about the sidelines with the two coaches and the manager helping to prod the team onward, he sat on the long, empty bench all by himself. So, naturally, we also referred to him as our "lonesome end."

Denny was so small we did not have the equipment to fit him properly. He drowned in his football gear. His oversized helmet— the smallest we had—bobbled around on his head when he went through calisthenics. The faceguard on the helmet protected one of his ears as often as it did his nose. The huge shoulder pads draped his small frame like two fluffy goose feather pillows, and sometimes you couldn't distinguish the shoulder from the head. His football pants looked like ruffled curtains that had been gathered around his waist, and the kneepads sank to his shins, midway between his knees and his ankles. His oversized cleats—again, the smallest we could find—curled upward at the toes. That spirited little guy was truly a sight to behold.

From Denny's perspective, size didn't count, and he strutted along the sidelines behaving like a giant. Being part of the team was all that mattered to him. He was the best team motivator we had ever known. He possessed enough team spirit to dish out an ample portion to each of the other players and still have plenty left over for himself. He had boundless faith in the team and his eagerness was contagious. The score could be 40–0 at halftime, and there he was, going around the locker room, pounding each player on the back, applauding the individual's efforts, encouraging him onward, and then standing at the door to give each player a strong butt-slap as the team headed back to the field. His never-give-up spirit made me wonder sometimes if he was aware of the score.

I suspected he also possessed the healthiest lungs with the loudest Tiger roar on the team. I often wondered how many times his battle cry had intimidated the hearing team in the next locker room. Sometimes I would stand in the hallway outside the locker rooms as the teams left for the field and study the faces and watch the eyes of the opposition players as they searched among our team for that "giant with that deafening roar." They would never have guessed it came from our four-footer.

If the outcome of football games were determined by the loudness of a roar or by a player's zeal, FOUR-SEVEN would have won every game for us that year.

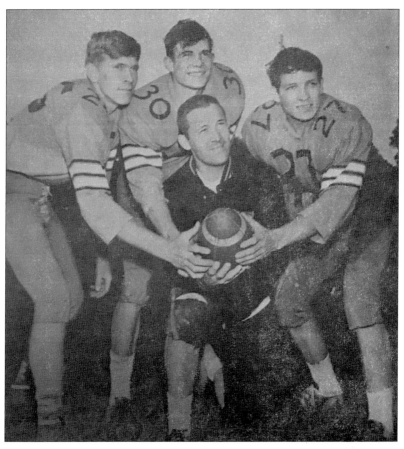

*Some of my football players. From left to right: Robert Schwisow,
Ken Eurek, and Terry Heidecker.*

TOM REMEMBERS . . .

The freshmen boys and I were operating the Kluge, the automatic platen press, when George Propp came in with the news. George was the high school science teacher and editor of the *Nebraska Journal*. He stopped by regularly to bring copy for the school publication, but on this particular morning he brought the news that would shock the nation. President John F. Kennedy had been assassinated in Dallas.

I shut off the press in a daze.

George and I shared the tragic news with the young boys in our presence and tried as best we could to respond to their barrage of "whys?" That was a question that swept the nation and the world and yet was never fully answered to anyone's satisfaction. Man's incomprehensible cruelty to man—why? Our nation had lost a promising young president. The boys were shocked and saddened, and each reacted to the news in a different way.

For young Tom, President Kennedy was his hero. He shared the president's love of the sea, a daring spirit, his boldness. And now his hero was gone. A skinny lad with black wavy hair on top of a long, narrow face, Tom was visibly shaken by the news like all of us.

After the class and I discussed the tragedy at length, and the boys had run out of questions and I had run out of answers, I tried to get the boys back to their work routines. But neither our hearts nor our minds were in it. When I looked around the room for Tom, I saw he had wandered over to the window. He stood looking out across the playground at Old Glory, fluttering at half-mast in the breeze. He remained there for a long time, and then I watched as he raised his right hand and placed it over his heart.

I had no idea what ran through his young mind at that moment. Perhaps it was his final salute to his hero and our fallen leader. Perhaps he was renewing his pledge to his flag and his country. Perhaps he was saying a prayer for a grieving family and nation.

Whatever was in Tom's mind, his gesture is forever frozen in my memory. Today, when I come across something related to President Kennedy, I see young Tom once again standing at the window, looking out at the flag, his hand over his heart trying to comprehend in his young mind a tragedy none of us will ever fully understand.

"GOOD LUCKY'S" SPECIAL CHARM

Strange as it may seem, when I taught at NSD, we had no sign for the expression "good luck." There was a sign for GOOD and a sign for LUCKY, but none for "luck" or the phrase "good luck." The sign LUCKY had at least two meanings with the difference depending on the facial expression and body language. When the kids signed LUCKY with an envious look on their face, a slight shake of their head and an "I-don't-believe-it" expression, they meant "I envy you," or "Gosh, you're soooo lucky!" If they used the "gee-whiz" surprised reaction and shook their hand in front of them for wow, then signed LUCKY, they were saying, "Wow, you're sooooo lucky!"

Typically, a signer signs GOOD then fingerspells L-U-C-K to express those good wishes to another person. But for the kids who used it so often—especially during football season—that was too cumbersome and slow, especially when everything was in motion, such as when the team was getting up to leave or boarding the bus or the bus was pulling out for a game on the road. So the team's young admirers invented their own speedy sign combination. They combined the two signs GOOD and LUCKY and out came the unique wish of GOOD LUCKY that, at least for me, would always have a special charm.

Translated into English, "good lucky" was a term that would send a nails-on-a-chalkboard shiver up an English teacher's spine. To this football coach, however, it had an exceptional meaning and GOOD LUCKY became a very popular sign used by the younger students during my last years as coach. And because it was their sign, I never had the heart to try to correct or change it. I argued—and convinced—myself that as they grew older, they would encounter enough language perfectionists along the way and learn the correct usage of "good luck." Why should I worry about that and spoil its unique meaning? Especially when it gave our team that little extra luck we always needed? In those days, during the football season, we required the team to dress well when we played away games. The school felt it was important that our team leave the best possible impression with the host schools. That meant that the boys wore white shirts and ties and jackets on away game days. As time passed, I noticed that the younger kids started dressing up on away game days, too. Puzzled about this, one day I stopped a little fellow named Clinton to question him.

"Why are you wearing a tie and jacket today?"

"You forgot?!" he signed to me, a startled expression on his face as he looked at me, the coach. "Today is an away game day!"

"Ohhhh!" I signed meekly.

So, as it happened, when the football team prepared to depart for their off-campus games, the younger kids, dressed to the nines like their heroes, would gather around the parked bus as the athletes boarded. The small fry would mingle with the players and wish each GOOD LUCKY. I would watch as the athletes beamed, thanked their young fans, and boarded the bus feeling very important, very special. I am sure the players felt, as I did, that there was a little extra measure of good luck in that special "good lucky" wish. As a coach who had gone through some pretty dismal seasons, who was I to quarrel with this fractured English version?

As our football fortunes improved, GOOD LUCKY became one of *my* favorite signed expressions! Although my coaching career ended many years ago, as I write this, I realize I still occasionally use this special expression today among my friends and professional colleagues to wish them that little "extra" luck.

LIFE AND FOOTBALLS TAKE FUNNY BOUNCES

In many ways, the game of football resembles the game of life. Football and life are both full of ups and downs, and our fortunes, like footballs, are always taking unusual bounces. Both are fraught with difficulties and frustrations and require much commitment and hard work before we can experience success. And no matter how hard you work, success is never guaranteed. But there are rewards and joy for those willing to make those kinds of commitments and who do not give up. As I was to learn as a coach on NSD's Booth Field, success is measured in many ways, and the boys and I learned together the true meaning of teamwork.

The year after we were wiped out with only nine players on our eight-man football team, an infusion of new players helped the NSD Tigers bounce back and post an amazing 6–2 record, one of the school's best. The next season the team set its goals even higher.

We beat Murdock, 39–7, in the season's opener. Ken, our quarterback, scored three touchdowns and caught a fifty-seven-yard pass from Cliff, our lineman-turned-fullback. Doug caught a thirty-five-yard touchdown pass from Ken, and Terry scampered forty-eight yards to pay dirt.

Our next opponent was Fort Calhoun, which had beaten us 55–26 the previous season. In this game, Ken scored seven touchdowns, including a seventy-five-yard punt return, and passed for another. He would have scored even more had I not taken him out of the game. Doug's younger brother taught himself how to drop-kick extra points and drop-kicked seven points in this game, setting a one-game school record, as we throttled Fort Calhoun, 63–13.

Our third game was against the very tough and much heavier West Kearney Vikings in the western part of the state. From the outset, the game was a cliff-hanger. During the game, Doug was hurt. He was knocked down and trampled on by the Viking's burly fullback. Assistant Coach Bryant and I ran onto the

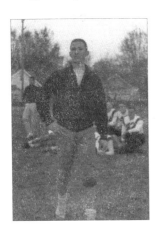

As a football coach.

field and checked him out for broken bones. Finding none, we pulled him up from the ground and helped him to the sidelines.

"I quit! I quit!" he signed angrily at me, his face contorted in pain as he limped off the field. "I'm not going back in there!" he signed, pointing his thumb over his shoulder in the direction of the skirmish. On the sidelines, he bent over, holding his stomach, and groaned.

Doug had been playing safety, the last man on defense. When all our other defenders had missed, Doug found himself all alone defending the goal post and staring at the Vikings' charging 200-pounds-plus, bullnecked fullback. How well I knew that very lonesome feeling. As a high school freshman, I, too, had been in his shoes. It is a terribly frightening and lonely place to be: it feels like standing in a pasture being charged by a mad bull.

Counting his uniform, pads, and throwing in his helmet and football shoes, Doug probably weighed a little more than half of what the fullback did. As the fullback rumbled toward him, Doug did what any other mortal player his size would do. He closed his eyes, bent his head down, stretched out his arms, and tried to make the tackle. Instead of skirting around Doug, the fullback saw him as a challenge and gamely bent low and plowed ahead. The fullback's helmet crashed into our little hero's stomach, knocking the wind out of him, along with—at that moment—all his football ambitions. In the process of tangling with

Doug, however, the fullback stumbled, lost his balance, and, with his legs flailing, plowed into the field! Doug had brought him down and prevented a touchdown!

Doug was a fierce competitor, and admittedly, I was surprised by his outburst. He didn't sound at all like the Doug I knew. Except for the unpleasant experience and getting the wind knocked out of him, he was otherwise unhurt. I put an arm over Doug's shoulder, and suddenly the action on the field became a blur. In Doug's place, I saw myself dressed in the MSD green and gold Eagle's uniform. I, too, was limping off the field. There was a lump on my leg the size of a tennis ball. I had received a direct kick in the shin. The pain had shot up to my stomach, which did several flip-flops before tightening into a knot. Suddenly, the game of football no longer held any appeal to me either. In that instant, I felt more like a chicken than an eagle. On the sidelines, I tapped Coach Baldridge on the shoulder and pointed at the painful lump. Coach bent down, took a close look at my injury, nodded his head in sympathy, then reassured me, "It'll be okay. You'll have to go back in. We have no center substitute." That was something I already knew but did not want to hear. As in life, when you get knocked down, you have no choice but to get back up. I knew well how Doug felt.

A commotion of shouting, flailing arms, and jumping on the sidelines caught my attention and brought me back to reality.

Our boys had recovered a fumble, and we had possession of the ball. The fortunes of football had once again turned in our favor. I, too, jumped with joy and shouted and turned to send in the offensive unit. When I looked at where Doug had stood moments before, the spot was empty. The brief rest had done him good. It had restored his confidence, rekindled his fighting spirit, and before I knew it, he was back on the playing field as determined as before.

We led in the fourth quarter by five meager points as the time on the clock slowly ran out. One touchdown by the Vikings and they would win the game.

The Vikings had the ball, and they started their goalward drive as the few remaining minutes on the clock ticked away slowly. The Vikings kept pushing our defense back as they moved closer and closer to the goal line. A touchdown seemed imminent. The year before, they had scored with only twenty seconds left on the clock to tie the game. I feared a repeat performance.

Their drive kept going, and we were not able to stop them. It was now fourth down, and they were two yards from the goal line with only a few seconds left on the clock. This was their last play, and it would determine the outcome of the game. We all knew that one little mistake, one missed tackle, and that was it. I braced for what was to come.

The Vikings' quarterback took the snap, turned around, and tossed the ball to his halfback. They had opted for an end run, and the halfback started toward the end zone. The Vikings' linemen executed their blocks almost perfectly, and one by one, our linemen fell or were blocked. Suddenly, one of our defensive backs dashed through an opening in the line, clashed with the halfback, and they fell. It was Ken. He nailed the runner two yards from the goal and saved the game. We went home with a 25–20 victory. The team and I sat on the bus all the way back to Omaha, dazed by the boys' determination and what had happened.

THE GAME WE *REALLY* WON

With that victory over West Kearney, our record stood at three wins and no losses. The excitement and anticipation of another winning season gripped the school. The players became more ambitious. They set their sights higher. There was talk of an undefeated season. The small fry started pushing that goal.

Prior to each game, the younger boys in the printshop, who were learning to hand-set type, started printing small cards on scrap paper with a simple message. The first week the cards read: "We want 1–0!" meaning, of course, they wanted a victory. The second week, the cards read, "We want 2–0!" and the third week, "We want 3–0!" and so on. Each week, as the season progressed, the number on the left side of those cards increased and the zero on the right remained the same. It was an exhilarating time for all of us. The boys distributed their cards to all the students, teachers, and staff members, and many pinned them on their clothes as a sign of support. The players got the message. School spirit soared.

The game with Brownell-Talbot (B-T), our rival across town, was played during a downpour. We had a superb passing attack, but the rain hampered it. It was hard enough to throw the football and catch it on the run without it being wet and slippery. B-T was a strong team and had an outstanding halfback.

From the outset, we had difficulty making our offense click. The downpour continued, and at halftime, we trailed by nine points. We needed two touchdowns to win. We were not only drenched to the bone but also drained of spirit. To make matters worse, as we slogged off the field to the locker room at halftime, we saw many of our fans get up and leave, adding to the gloom. They considered the outcome a foregone conclusion and saw no reason to sit through the soaking second half. Our hopes of an undefeated season were being washed away in the rain.

We were still nine points behind going into the final quarter. I stood on the sidelines, outwardly a picture of calm. Under the heavy football parka, however, my nerves did somersaults. Pessimism steamrolled me.

With three minutes left on the clock, we got possession of the ball but soon found ourselves with eight yards to go on our own forty-yard line. I told Ken to punt, hoping that with the rain, we might recover a fumble or stop B-T in their own territory and get the ball back.

The boys lined up in punt formation with Ken as the kicker. But Ken and Doug had other ideas. They had decided to gamble and to put all the stakes on that one play. Instead of punting, Ken went for the bomb—a long, surprise pass, on our own forty-yard line. That gamble shocked me; neither B-T nor I had expected it. If it failed, it would give B-T possession of the ball and put them in an easy scoring position. I watched Doug scamper down the field alone, and I saw Ken take the snap, run to the backfield, lean backward, and loft the ball in a long, high arc. The other team, expecting a punt, had only three defenders in their backfield. All eyes followed that arc as the ball spiraled and wobbled in the rain. By the time Ken let go of the pass, Doug had run past two of the defenders, who obviously thought the pass was a fluke, and had the third defender chasing him. The ball came down in Doug's outstretched hands with a plop and a splash. The last defender was out of range, and Doug crossed the goal line untouched. We had scored! The few remaining fans and the boys on the sidelines went wild with joy. It was unbelievable, but we were still two points behind, and we needed either a field goal or one more touchdown to win the game.

Precious little time remained on the clock, and with us kicking off, it would give B-T possession of the ball. That would give them an important advantage, and naturally, they would hang on to that ball for dear life and run out the clock.

Although I am a Christian, I never believed in praying for victory. In sports competitions, I had always felt that God should remain neutral and let us mortals compete on our own merits. I always prayed instead that each player would do his best, that none would get seriously hurt, and whatever the outcome of the game, we, as a team, would walk off the field as proudly as we had walked on to it, each with the satisfaction of knowing we had given it our all. At that moment, however, I broke my self-imposed rule and sent up an earnest, urgent, silent plea for help. I was sure God would understand. We had come so far, I argued, we just couldn't lose this one! I felt the boys had rightfully earned a little extra help, and since the rain was in B-T's favor, surely we qualified for a little trade-off.

The teams lined up for the kickoff. We decided to go for an onside kick where the ball is bounced on the ground instead of kicked high in the air. A football is harder to catch when it is bouncing every which way on the ground. Once it crosses the ten yards separating the two teams, it becomes a "free" ball and belongs to whichever team pounces on it first. This is the best chance the kicking team has to get the ball back. But the ball would be in their territory, and we had to get to it fast before one of their players did. Then maybe, just maybe, with the few seconds left on the clock, we could score and win the game. That was the play B-T expected.

We kicked the ball, it bounced and skidded on the wet field, crossed the ten-yard zone, and plopped into the waiting hands of one of their linesmen. But then it slipped through his hands onto the ground. Two of our players knocked him out of the way and pounced on it. We had gotten possession of the ball! We now had one slim, final chance to win. I looked heavenward and nodded my thanks. The game scene and mood changed dramatically. Our successful bomb pass and now the quick recovery of the onside kick bowled over the B-T team. These back-to-back plays had knocked the fight out of our opponents and caused last-minute panic in their ranks while igniting our boys. We had enough time for just one play, one last chance. We called our last time-out and Ken, Coach Bryant, and I discussed our options and agreed on the strategy. We decided to go for a pass to Doug.

The teams lined up facing each other. Ken took the snap and ran to the backfield to pass, well-protected by our line, but B-T had anticipated a pass play. They had Doug and all our other receivers well-covered. Ken couldn't find an open receiver, so he chose the only remaining option: he decided to run for it. He zig-zagged down the field toward the distant goal posts. He dodged one tackler after another. Several hearts—mine included—must have skipped several beats during that run. As Ken neared the goal, B-T's last defender challenged him. The tackler narrowly missed and Ken scored. The clock expired, the whistle blew, the fans and players roared. The game was over. The final score was 39–34 in our favor. We had made an unbelievable comeback and squeaked by. We hugged, back-slapped each other, shouted until we were hoarse, and jubilantly trod off the soggy field. It was still raining, but suddenly none of us felt wet any more.

The following Monday morning, Dallas, one of the teachers, approached me with a long, sympathetic face, shook his head, and signed sadly, "Sorry about last Friday." He had been one of those fans who had given up hope, left at halftime, and was too dejected to read the Sunday sports page.

"Why?" I asked.

"Too bad you lost," he responded.

"Lost?" I asked. "No, we won!"

"You won?!?" He looked stunned. "You really won?"

"Yes," I told him, nodding my head happily. "That was a game we *really* won!"

ON BEING A WINNER

The game with Malcolm High School was another close encounter. To raise the stakes and make it more exciting, it fell on Friday the thirteenth. We recovered a fumble on our own two-yard line and scored with only thirty seconds left to squeak out of that one. Doug caught three touchdown passes and Bob ran for two touchdowns. Cliff led the defense with thirteen tackles. It was another hair-raiser that ended 39–32 in our favor.

The following week, we beat Monroe High School, 51–38.

In the game with Craig, once again, we had to come from behind in the fourth quarter to win. Ken made two touchdowns in the final four minutes to pull us out of that one, 32–19.

By now, the cards our young Benjamin Franklins were printing and distributing on campus read, "We Want 8–0" and NSD had a few nervous people around. The final game of the season was with Waterloo, our strongest opponent and the pregame favorite. It was a night game, and because it was after work hours, it drew a large crowd. Many members of the Deaf community, the school's alumni, parents, and teachers attended. It turned out to be another thriller.

We were taking a season record of seven wins and no losses into this contest and, understandably, all of us were on pins and needles. This game would make or break the team's goal of an undefeated season. From the very beginning, it was a hard-fought contest. By halftime, the score stood deadlocked, 0–0. It was obvious that the boys were as wired as the coaches. We were playing too cautiously. Somehow, we had to get over our obsession with an undefeated season and hit the playing field full throttle. Unless we got into the game mentally, we would let our own nervousness beat us. We had to start playing the brand of football we were accustomed to, or we were going to experience a real heartbreaker.

In the locker room at halftime, I flicked the lights and waved my hand to get the boys' attention. I didn't know what I was going to do, but I had to think of something. "Well . . ." I signed to the boys, trying to appear as nonchalant as I could, "We've come a long way, don't you think? We've had a great year, right?" All the boys nodded in agreement.

"Question," I signed, "Did you realize that in another thirty minutes football will be finished? Next Monday, you will send your uniforms to the laundry, and we will put away all the football gear. This will be the last season for some of you." YOU FIN-

ISH. YOU FINISH. YOU FINISH, I signed, pointing to individual players who were playing their last game.

I stopped to let what I had said sink in. The boys eyed me, wondering what I was up to.

"Like you," I continued, "I came here tonight hoping for an undefeated record . . . 8–0." I paused again and took a swallow. "We all want 8–0. The students, the teachers, Coach Bryant, and I want 8–0. You want 8–0." I paused again and waited a little while. "But . . . I just want you to know," I signed slowly, " . . . if we go home tonight with 7–1, Coach Bryant and I will still be bursting with pride." Coach Bryant and I looked at each other and nodded our heads in agreement.

The boys were quiet for a while as they thought about what I had just said, then it registered on their faces. The idea of abandoning our goal of an undefeated season upset them and ticked them off. One face after the other changed from a look of anxiety and anticipation to one of anger and steel. I had insulted them! I had compromised our season's goal, and they were hopping mad. I had—I hoped—diverted their thoughts away from the jitters back to the moment. Their old fight began to bubble again, and, one by one, they raised clenched fists in the air and yelled. Then, collectively, they let out a war-whoop that was probably heard clear across that little town. They were not ready to settle for a loss . . . not yet.

Following the halftime break, the team charged out of the locker room with a roar that reminded me of FOUR-SEVEN's a few years previously. Surely, the Waterloo team next door heard it and got the message.

The kickoff took place, and both teams played conservative football to prevent the other from scoring. Late in the third quarter, Ken connected with Doug for a fifteen-yard touchdown pass. Ken made the extra point and we were up 7–0. On our next possession, however, Waterloo intercepted a pass and ran it back seventy yards for a touchdown. That stunned us. They failed, however, to convert their extra point, and we led by a 7–6 margin. We had to keep going, but we couldn't afford to take any risky moves. One little mistake could cost us the game.

In the fourth quarter, we ran into some serious trouble. Three times we found ourselves in a fourth-down situation. We could punt and give up the ball or gamble and run the ball, hoping for a first down and retaining possession of the ball. Three times we took the risk and ran the ball. Three times we made a first down. Throughout that quarter, it was touch and go.

Late in the quarter, Ken scored on a pass interception, but we failed with the point conversion, giving us a 13–6 lead. Waterloo could still tie the game. They took possession of the ball and started their march down the field, but our defense tightened, and we stopped their drive. Once again, we took possession of the ball and started running out the clock. At long last, we had the ball on Waterloo's thirty-yard line with twenty-five seconds remaining on the clock. One more play, and the game would be over.

To my surprise, Ken called a time-out. I was puzzled because there was no reason for a time-out. All that remained to do was kill the ball, and the game—and season—would be over. Ken knew that. There was no reason to consult with the coaches.

I watched as Dick, our manager, ran out to the boys huddled on the field lugging his heavy water bucket, towels flapping over his shoulders. I saw Ken trotting toward me on the sidelines. As he approached, I could see behind his faceguard that familiar, broad smile. He came up to me, shook my hand, winked, slapped Coach Bryant on the shoulder then turned around and jogged back to the huddle!

Not a word was said. But our eyes had met, and the message was clear. The season was ours! The boys' teamwork, togetherness, and belief in themselves and in each other had paid off. We were 8–0. We had made it! Our dream of an undefeated season had come true.

Ken had called a time-out because he wanted to be the first to acknowledge our success. That fleeting moment with my quarterback on the sidelines just seconds before the conclusion of that season was my greatest thrill in sports. Back on the field,

Ken killed the ball. The gun went off and bedlam followed. The team and fans went wild. The fans ran shouting, flailing their arms onto the field to congratulate the players. There was yelling, jumping, bear-hugging, backslapping, and kissing. The NSD Tigers, their coaches, and the fans became one huge, happy mass of joy.

We had done it! We had racked up the school's first undefeated football season! But more important than an undefeated season was that each player had proven to himself, his family, and the school community that he was a winner. That experience taught each of them that with a little luck and a lot of grit, they could do anything they set their hearts to.

POSTSCRIPT TO THE LAST SEASON

For some of us, the Waterloo game was a bittersweet ending. Much later that night, after Coach Bryant and I had been carried off the field on the players' shoulders and ceremoniously doused in the showers, after most of the exhilaration of the evening had died down, the happy NSD fans had finally departed, and the boys had taken their showers and donned their street clothes, I blinked the lights for attention. I had some important news to tell them.

This was our last meeting as a football team. I had news that I had been holding onto for more than a month. What a nasty way to end such a wonderful season, I thought. The news would be released on the school campus on Monday. I wanted the boys to be the first to hear it, and I wanted them to get it directly from me.

I watched as the team came together and began to quiet down. As I looked at each face, I recalled the close relationship I had with each individual, either as his teacher or coach or both. How fortunate I felt to have had the opportunity to work with such a wonderful bunch of youngsters—to get to know them personally, to share their outlook on life, and their hopes and ambitions. I hoped, in some way, I had made a positive contribution to each of their dreams.

Their happy, excited faces looked back at me expectantly, curious, waiting.

I took a long swallow and announced: "This is my last year at NSD." I signed rapidly, fighting to control my emotions, "Mrs. Gannon and I will be leaving Nebraska this summer."

After much personal agony and many sleepless nights, I had decided to accept a new position at Gallaudet College in Washington, DC. I had been offered the dual role of becoming the first full-time executive secretary of the Gallaudet College Alumni Association and the director of the new Alumni Relations Program. Rosalyn had accepted a position as an art teacher at the Kendall School, an elementary school on the same campus.

The happy looks on the boys' faces quickly vanished. They were jarred out of their happy dreams back to the reality of life. The season was over. Their eyes conveyed shock, hurt, and puzzlement. The expected barrage of "whys?" quickly followed.

The team set a new school record for the longest winning streak in the school's history. The NSD Tigers became the first eight-man football team among the national schools for the deaf to post an undefeated record. One local sports writer described the season as ". . . one of the most noteworthy athletic feats in the school's history."

Ken was named to Art Kruger's All-America eleven-man football team in *The Deaf American* and Doug made honorable mention. Ken led the state in scoring and was selected to the All-State eight-man football team by the *Omaha World-Herald*. Doug set a three-season NSD reception record. I was named "Coach of the Year" by the Omaha WOW-TV station.

Six of the boys—including Doug and "Pizza" Eddie—became printers. Four of the players went on to college and two to technical schools. Mike got a job in the home improvement business, RS, Bob, John, Leon, and Richard secured work in the manufacturing, home construction, and meat-processing fields. Pat returned to the farm. Cliff went on disability from a neck injury. Darrel's life ended tragically. Terry and Dick moved out of

I received a football from Kenneth Eurek and our football team at my farewell dinner, 1968.

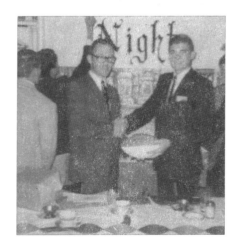

state. Alan got a job with the Nebraska State Roads Department. After college, Ken became a teacher and coach at the Colorado School for the Deaf and the Blind, and Larry Johnson, one of the printers, raised sheep on the side. When I met him some years later, he told me he had been elected vice president of the Nebraska Sheep Growers Association. A few are unemployed and I've lost contact with the rest.

Rosalyn and I left Nebraska one week after school closed that summer, though part of us will remain there forever.

PART THREE

BECOMING PARENTS

Language for the Eye

Hold a tree in the palm of your hand,

or topple it with a crash.

Sail a boat on finger waves,

or sink it with a splash.

From your fingers tips see a frog leap,

at a passing butterfly.

The word becomes the picture in this language for the eyes.

Follow the sun from rise to set,

or bounce it like a ball.

Catch a fish in a fishing net.

or swallow it, bones and all.

Make traffic scurry, or airplanes fly,

and people meet and part.

The word becomes the action in this language of the heart.

—Dorothy Miles

Dorothy Miles (1931–1993) became deaf when she was eight. She received her elementary education in Wales and enrolled in Gallaudet College (now University) in 1957. Following Gallaudet, she became involved with renowned ASL poets Clayton Valli and Ella Mae Lentz and wrote "Language for the Eye," mixing her native British Sign Language and her new ASL into poetry.

INTRODUCTION

In the early 1970s, the Gannons became parents to a son and a daughter. As Deaf parents of hearing children, they navigated all the trials and joys of raising a family along with the unique communication challenges, problem-solving opportunities, and comical situations arising from Deaf–hearing relations. Jeff, born in 1971, and Christine, born in 1973, both learned ASL as infants and toddlers, while also learning English. As parents, Jack and Rosalyn emphasized appreciation for both languages. Their filled-with-books home and Jack's prolific writing demonstrated their love of the written word, while all conversation was in ASL.

Changes in communications access developed along with the Gannon family. New technology such as teletypes (TTYs) and television captioning made it possible for Jack and Rosalyn to watch television news and programs, though many were not captioned at the time. Through public performances and media, society was becoming more aware of Deaf people as a cultural and linguistic group, and this would impact the Gannons's sense of pride and identity as a Deaf and hearing family.

WE MOVE TO A "QUIET" NEIGHBORHOOD

In 1969, several months after we had moved to the Washington, DC, area, Rosalyn and I began house hunting. We had a nice apartment and we had some very good neighbors and friends, but neither of us relished living in an apartment. I missed my workshop, yard work, and the freedom of puttering in the outdoors, and Rosalyn missed a large kitchen and a sewing room. More importantly, we were expecting our first child and wanted to establish a home and roots in the community.

After months and months of weekend searching and visiting houses on the market, we finally found one that we both liked in Silver Spring, Maryland. It was in a suburban neighborhood near good schools and a nice shopping center with a supermarket not too far away. An older house with a brick exterior, Rosalyn liked the kitchen layout and the house floor plan. It had a large backyard, a sunny garden spot, and a basement area that would make an ideal workshop. Of course, it cost more than we really wanted to pay, but we were both happy with it. The only negative thing about it was that it was at least a thirty-minute drive from where we worked.

One day after work, we made another appointment with the real estate agent to take one last look at the house and discuss the price before making an offer. We had just completed the final tour of the house with the agent and were debating with ourselves in sign language whether or not we could afford the asking price and monthly payments. The agent, who knew no sign language, could sense our apprehension. With a pad in one hand and pen in the other, he kept trying very hard to convince us of the wonderful opportunity we had before us. He would take us through different parts of the house, point out something with the pen, then quickly scribble a positive note on the pad and vigorously shake his head in the affirmative to visibly emphasize his point.

"This house is very well built!" he wrote as he pounded his fist against the wall for added emphasis. "The previous owners were a retired, elderly couple who took good care of the house," he scribbled, the palm of his hand sweeping around the room. "It is a steal at the asking price!" he went on, pounding his fist on the pad to stress his point. We nodded at each comment to indicate that we were listening as our eyes gazed longingly about our dream home. We tried to not give away our desire for and anxiety about the house because we knew that that would make the price negotiation harder.

At the end of the tour, the three of us walked out the front door and stood in the front yard, viewing the beautiful surrounding homes with their neatly kept lawns and the tree-lined street. As the agent looked about the neighborhood, he thought of another sales pitch, and not wanting to miss a single opportunity to close the deal, he held up his pen to catch our attention and quickly scribbled on the pad. Then he pointed the pen down the street in a circular motion around the neighborhood and showed us the pad where he had written: "What's more, it's a very quiet neighborhood!!!" The words "quiet neighborhood" were underlined for emphasis. Obviously, he had forgotten we were deaf.

Rosalyn and I were amused and smiled as we read the comment and looked at each other. The realtor looked pleased and displayed an air of satisfaction with his clever last sales pitch, not realizing the irony of what he had just said. I turned to him, circled those two words he had underlined repeatedly, and wrote: "That's just what we need!"

The agent read the response momentarily puzzled, then the smile on his face vanished as he suddenly realized that in his enthusiasm to make a sale he had forgotten that we were deaf.

"Ohhh . . ." we lipread him utter as he let out a deflated sigh when he realized the irony of what he had just written. A puzzled look appeared on his face indicating he was wondering whether he had made a blunder with that silly comment. He elected not to say anything further and made a feeble attempt at a smile. Fortunately for the agent, Rosalyn and I thought his remark and the situation were both amusing and laughed. The agent soon joined us in the laughter about his unthinking, over-zealous attempt at a final sales pitch.

We bought the house, and it wasn't long before we learned that it really was a quiet neighborhood! Then, Rosalyn experienced those rumbling trucks in the night.

RUMBLING TRUCKS IN THE NIGHT

One morning not long after we moved to our quiet neighborhood, Rosalyn told me she had felt a big truck rumble by during the night. I looked at her skeptically. I didn't believe it. I argued that our residential area, away from a main traffic thoroughfare, was no place for big trucks. While she agreed, she insisted there had been a loud, rumbling noise and that it felt like a big truck. We assumed it must have been something else and let the matter drop.

Some days later at breakfast, Rosalyn again mentioned feeling the vibrations of a rumbling truck. She was sure that she had felt a large truck pass on the street right outside our house, she explained. She was positive that it had occurred. It was so heavy, she recalled, that it seemed to shake the house. I was puzzled, but still full of doubt.

"Did you get up and go to the window and check?" I asked.

"No," she said, "I was too lazy. I wanted to sleep," and once again the matter was dropped.

Sometime later, she woke up feeling that strange vibration again. At first, she thought she had been dreaming, but on waking up, knew she wasn't. Quickly she got up and hurried to the front bay window and looked out. To her surprise there was not a single moving vehicle in sight. Only the tree branches and electric wires swayed and danced in the wind, making the street lights blink.

She crawled back into bed and lay there, puzzled, then curled up next to me and was soon fast asleep. Suddenly, the vibrations woke her again. She raised her head from the pillow and forced her sleepy eyes open. She was determined to find the cause of that noise. The moonlight shone through our window and she looked about the room and bed.

I was asleep on my back, my mouth agape. She rested her hand and arm on my chest and felt the vibration. It turned out that I was the "rumbling truck in the night." I was snoring.

BABY-CRY SIGNALS

We were ready for our firstborn, Jeff, when he came home from the hospital. At least, we thought so.

Older parents had shared with us their anxiety and experience with babies. Many of the couples told us of the improvisations they made to cope with being unable to hear the baby's cry during the night. Some mothers would place the baby's crib next to their side of the bed and sleep with one hand and arm in the crib to feel the baby's movement and cries. Other couples told us how they slept with the baby between them so they both could feel the infant. One mother recalled waking one night to find the baby missing and realized that the father was sleeping on top of the infant! Fortunately, the baby was unharmed. Others told us that their family doctor had advised them not to worry and to let the baby cry during the night. It was good for developing healthy lungs, he said.

We were a bit luckier. We entered parenthood during the age of better technology, and that gave us more confidence that we would be prepared for Jeff's every whim . . . almost. How unwittingly true that turned out to be!

Like all typical parents, we had set up Jeff's room and his new crib weeks before his arrival. Jeff's dresser, on which I had painted clown faces on each drawer with the drawer handles as noses, was ready. Rosalyn had made new curtains to match. On top of the dresser was the baby powder, the baby oil, cotton swabs, and all the other essentials that go with the baby trade. Next to it and in the closet were stacks and stacks of cloth and disposable diapers. What a blessing they turned out to be.

The crib had one distinct difference from most other cribs. Wired to one end of it was an electronic device. We had acquired a homemade baby-cry signal from deaf friends whose children were grown. Since neither of us could hear the baby cry, we needed a way to know when the little fellow was unhappy or

Jeff in his new bedroom.

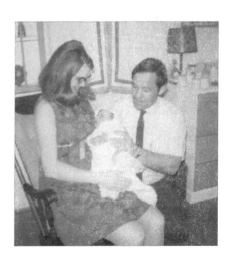

uncomfortable, and this cry signal was built to do just that. This thing consisted of a microphone attached to the baby's crib and wired to a relay system under it. A wire ran from the relay system to a lamp in our bedroom. When the baby cried, the microphone picked up the sound, and the relay system made the light in our bedroom flash, waking us up.

It was a great invention, really, a great device, but things did not initially work out quite as we expected. With babies, do they ever?! The first several nights, we learned that the volume on the relay system was taking longer to adjust to the proper noise level than we realized. The microphone was unsophisticated and responded to all kinds of noises. Being new parents, when the light flashed, we were out of bed and on our feet in an instant, usually bumping into each other in the darkness as we raced for the

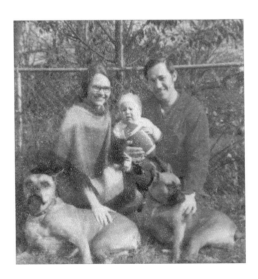

Family picture with our two dogs, Suzie and Dixie, 1971.

baby's room. But, as explained, the unsophisticated microphone had a tendency to pick up all kinds of noises. When Jeff cried, the microphone worked well. But it also worked when a car with a loud muffler went by outside, sending us off to the baby's room only to find him sleeping peacefully. When a noisy truck passed by outside, we repeated our performance. When the garbage collectors came early in the morning and dropped the trash cans or when a door slammed, the light flashed. After repeating the process a while it became a bit tiresome, to put it mildly, and by the end of the first week, I noticed that our response time had deteriorated badly. It wasn't doing much for our sleep, either. This lack of sleep puzzled some of my coworkers. When they witnessed me dragging myself into the office in the morning in a rumpled suit or with shoulders stooped and heavy bags under my eyes, they wondered visibly and out loud: "I thought only hearing parents lost sleep over crying babies during the night."

After much trial and error, we finally got the sound system adjusted about right so that the microphone would ignore most outside noises and only picked up Jeff's wail. We also learned how to distinguish between the frequency of the blinking lights from his crying and from other noises. Our nights settled down and our sleep improved until we entered the second phase of the experience.

Some months after Jeff's arrival, he started standing up in his crib, and he learned that when he rattled its side, one of us always responded. So, any time he wanted attention, he would shake the side of the crib. This started our second battle with the baby-cry signal, and it lasted until Jeff was old enough to move to his own bed. By that time, a newcomer, Christy, had arrived and taken over the light-flashing chores.

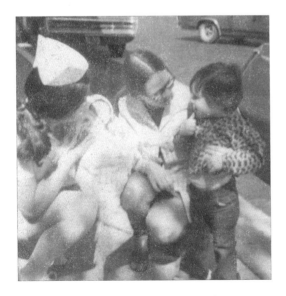

Jeff meets his new baby sister, Christine (see Jeff's sign GIRL*), May 2, 1973.*

LIVING WITH AND WITHOUT SOUND

Growing up as hearing children in a family with deaf parents requires improvisation on the kids' part as well as ours. Our house, like most of the homes of our deaf friends, is wired with a special light-flashing system. When someone calls us on the telephone or rings the doorbell, the house lights blink on and off. At night we are the only people in the neighborhood who send out a signal to the neighbors every time we have a visitor or receive a telephone call.

So perhaps it was only natural that the first sign our children learned was "light"—each time the house lights blinked, Rosalyn would make the sign for "lights blinking on and off," and both Jeff and Christy were about ten months old each when they began using that sign. LIGHTS BLINKING ON OFF they would sign with their tiny hands when the doorbell or the telephone rang. As they grew, they picked up other signs naturally. We observed with interest as their signing skills went through stages. First were the "baby signs"—comparable to baby babbling. The sign for "mother," for instance, is all five fingers spread out and the thumb placed on the chin. But small babies don't have that kind of hand coordination, so they often point to the chin with just the index finger.

As Jeff and Christy developed their signing skills, they went through periods of heavy reliance on fingerspelling (because they did not know enough signs). They began picking up more and more signs and eventually they struck a better balance of signs and fingerspelling.

They progressed through periods of baby signs, sloppy and careless, to more clarity and fluidity as they grew older. We encouraged both their speech and sign language development and we avoided being overly critical of wrong signs. We watched with pride as their sign language developed naturally—as it does with most offspring of deaf parents—and they picked up many sign language idioms and slang.

Rosalyn has often told me that she thinks deaf mothers have to work twice as hard as hearing mothers. "What do you mean?" I asked the first time she said this.

"There's more legwork involved," she explained. Being more visually acute without reliance on sound, the deaf mother must check on small children regularly to be sure that everything is okay. When Jeff was about two years old, he loved to play hide-and-seek. One day Rosalyn put Jeff in bed to nap and went downstairs to iron. When she went to check on Jeff, he was not in his bed. She looked throughout the house, thinking that he was playing hide-and-seek, but she couldn't find him. She began to panic.

"Jeff! Jeff!" she shouted. He didn't appear. She looked in each closet, and under each bed. Jeff was nowhere to be seen. She was becoming very upset when she glanced out the window overlooking the backyard and saw him prancing around with the dog. He had sneaked out behind her back, managed to open the glass sliding door, and gone romping in the backyard.

Another trick Jeff liked to play on his mother was when she vacuumed the house. He would slip up behind her and unplug the cord. The little rascal would sit back and watch and laugh

Jeff and Christine at Christmastime, 1973.

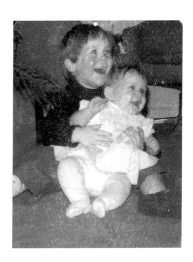

with glee when his mother finally discovered why her vacuum was not working after several passes over the carpet.

The kids learned early on that when they were playing outside and we were nearby but not watching them, they couldn't yell: "Hey Mom, hey Dad, watch me!" They had to stop whatever they were doing, run over to where we were, tap us on the arm to get our attention, and then run back to where they were and repeat what they were doing while we watched. Or they could command each other: "Get Mommy!" or "Get Daddy!"

Similarly, they knew they couldn't call for us when they needed help. One day when she was three years old, Christy discovered Jeff's toy handcuffs and accidentally handcuffed herself to a table leg in the living room. She couldn't get loose. Usually, she would have yelled for Jeff to "get Mommy!" but Jeff was at school, and no amount of shouting was going to do her any good. It was on a routine check that Rosalyn found Christy sitting there on the floor, handcuffed to the leg, tears streaming down her cheeks. After that experience, Christy never played with the handcuffs again.

Stomping a foot on the floor, pounding a fist on the table or slapping it with the palm of the hand, flickering the room lights, waving a hand, or tapping a family member on the shoulder are all normal attention-getting strategies in a normal deaf household. Sometimes, they can be a bit habit-forming. One summer, after an extended visit to my home in Missouri, my family got into the habit of tapping either Rosalyn or me on the shoulder whenever they wanted our attention. After we had departed, the practice lingered on a while; some hearing family members would tap other hearing family members on the shoulder to get their attention, provoking this tart reply: "Hey, you don't have to tap me on the shoulder—I can hear you!"

One thing our kids had to learn was that we could call them vocally but they couldn't call us. Likewise, when one deaf spouse wants the other deaf spouse, we don't call—we go searching. If you don't know where the other person is at the moment, it can sometimes result in a time-consuming house search. After one such exhaustive search for me, Rosalyn found me on my hands and knees organizing a basement storage closet. She leaned back against the door jamb, held her wrist to her forehead, and sighed. "Thank God we don't have a larger house!" Other times when I was working outside and unwittingly moved around the house, she would chase me from behind trying to catch my attention.

While we did not like to have to ask, Jeff and Christy had to interpret for us sometimes in many different situations. Their use of sign language impressed many hearing people, but not most of our deaf friends who viewed such development as natural. Hearing people would look on in amazement as they spoke and watched our small tots convert their spoken words into rapid finger and hand movements. Then these people would watch us nod our heads in understanding or see us respond. They would look at the kids, shake their heads in wonderment and say, "They sign so well!" We would smile and nod our heads in acknowledgment of their kindness and laugh inwardly, knowing that they had not the least idea what the kids were signing.

By encouraging our children's communication skills, we wanted them to feel comfortable in both worlds—theirs and ours. We knew they would learn all about the hearing world in school and from their friends, so we assumed the responsibility of introducing them to the world of deaf people. In the process they met and interacted with our deaf friends, and they learned about deaf people, our interests, our achievements, our culture, and our history.

Before Jeff and Christy started school, we cautioned them to expect some teasing from their peers because we were "different." When Jeff was in kindergarten, Rosalyn volunteered to speak to his class. She brought an interpreter with her so she could talk to the students and respond to their questions. She did the same thing with Christy's class, and the teacher invited her back for several years to speak to other classes. The young students expressed a keen interest in her talks, and some of them even learned to fingerspell afterward.

One day at school, Christy was trying to explain to a student that her parents were deaf. The little student did not understand, of course, and the following conversation ensued:

Student: "Why are your parents deaf?"

Christy: "Because they can't hear."

Student: "Why can't they hear?"

Christy: "Because they are deaf!" Realizing she was getting nowhere and then as an afterthought, she added, "Their ears are broken."

Student: "Oh."

During dinner one night, Jeff told us that one of the boys made fun of him during recess because his parents were deaf. We touched each other's knees under the table. We had been expecting and dreading this moment. "What did you say, Jeff?" we asked.

"Oh," signed Jeff, not showing the least bit of concern, "I asked him if his Mom and Dad used two languages and he said no."

Sometimes we unwittingly do things or make noises that embarrass the kids. One day near dinnertime, Christy turned to me, looked up, and admonished: "Daddy, your stomach is growling!" Another time, I mispronounced a word with which I was unfamiliar. Christy shook her head sideways and with a look of exasperation on her face, put her hands on her waist, and then scolded me: "Daddy! Daddy! You're saying it all wrong!"

One day when Rosalyn and Jeff were on their way to the grocery store, Jeff turned to his mother and said, "No offense, Mom. Please do not use your voice at the store."

Both Rosalyn and I had grown up with dogs, so it was only a matter of time following our wedding before we acquired a boxer. When the children arrived, Dixie was in the twilight of her years. Her black mask had turned gray, and she suffered from arthritis and a bad back, but she welcomed the children in the family like an affectionate nanny. However, Christy's arrival created one problem. When Rosalyn called "Dixie," Christy would come. "What do you want, Mommy?" Christy would ask. "I was calling Dixie," her mother would respond. At other times Rosalyn would call "Christy," and Dixie would come into the room, her ears perked up, and a "you called for me?" look on her face.

These coincidences puzzled Rosalyn, and it was not until Dixie had died, and we had gotten a new boxer puppy that we figured out what caused the confusion. The family was trying to decide on a name for the new puppy, and each time we found a name we liked, Christy asked her mother to shout it. Rosalyn and I thought that strange until we realized that Christy wanted a name that did not sound like hers. That was how we learned about the mix-up. We named the new puppy Lady.

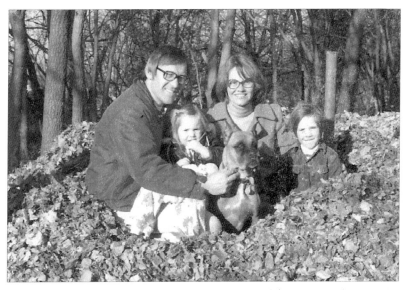

Family with Dixie, fall 1976.

JEFF PROVIDES A CROWNING MOMENT TO OUR LIVES

Jeff was five years old and had just started school when we got the announcement about the school's open house; neither Rosalyn nor I had looked forward to attending. We knew from past experience that it would be an "all look and little comprehension" situation since no attempt was made in those days to provide interpreters and involve deaf parents. But Rosalyn had argued how important it was for Jeff that we attend. I knew she was right, so I took the morning off from work to accompany her.

We entered the classroom, tiptoed to one side of the room, stood along the wall with other proud parents, and watched. The teacher looked up as we came in, smiled, and nodded her head in our direction, acknowledging our arrival. She knew we were deaf. We nodded and smiled back. The children noticed their teacher looking at the door and all turned to look at us. That's when Jeff saw us and that's when we knew that our decision to come was the right one. His face lit up like a Christmas tree. He stood up and pointed at us and told his class in voice and sign, "That's my Mommy and Daddy!"

The class storytelling period had just begun. The teacher gathered her twenty young charges about her in a semicircle on the carpet and began telling a Mother Goose story. We looked on knowing what she was doing, but not following what she was saying. Suddenly, Jeff turned around and looked at us and then back at his teacher who was speaking. He knew we did not understand what she was saying. He got up and walked over and stood next to the teacher. We were puzzled. We had not noticed the teacher call him, and the teacher, also puzzled, looked at him standing next to her. Then with his small hands and tiny fingers Jeff began "interpreting" and telling us as best he could what the teacher was saying.

He didn't realize it, of course, but for us, his thoughtful gesture was a crowning moment in his deaf parents' lives.

CHRISTY WISHES WE COULD HEAR

"I wish you could hear!" three-year-old Christy signed as she mouthed the words, and her face began to quiver. She was on the verge of tears.

"Why?" her mother and I asked almost simultaneously, glancing at each other in surprise and wondering what had caused the outburst. We had stopped at Aunt Sarah's Pancake House on our way to North Carolina to visit Rosalyn's parents. As the waitress approached our table with a bright smile and a cheery good morning greeting, Rosalyn and I had both acknowledged her friendly greeting with smiles and nods of our heads without uttering a word. We ordered our breakfast and the waitress left. Christy had heard the waitress's friendly welcome, but had heard no response from us, and thinking we had not noticed, had become upset.

Rosalyn looked at Christy and asked again, "Why do you wish we could hear?"

"Just because . . . just because . . ." Christy said and started to hiccup as tears welled up in her eyes. Her mother prodded for an answer, and Christy fidgeted in her chair. Finally she said, "The waitress talked to you and you and Daddy did not answer."

"Oh . . ." responded her mother. "That's true. We did not hear her, but we saw the smile on her face, and we smiled back. Didn't you see us smile? A smile is another way to greet people. You don't have to talk all the time."

"Oh . . ." said Christy. That hadn't occurred to her, and like most hearing-oriented people, she had only heard what went on and had not seen what had happened. "Ohhh . . ." she said again, visibly relieved. She turned her attention to a game on the table and the matter was forgotten. It was the first and only time Christy ever expressed a concern about our being deaf.

STUCK IN THE BATHROOM

When the children were very small, we had a rule. When one had to go to the potty, the other stayed within ear shot so that when the bathroom-goer was done, the other would know when to go and fetch Mom or Dad to do the "paper chores" and help pull up the pants.

"Christeee! Get Mommy!" Jeff would yell. Or, "Jeffff! Jeffff! Get Daddy!" Christy would shout. Then, the one not on the potty would run up to us, poke us in the leg and sign, "Christy wants you!" or "Jeff wants you!"

The system worked great until the day Jeff wandered off out of ear shot, leaving Christy sitting there on the potty. "Jeffff! Get Mommy! Jeffff! JEFFFFFFFF! Get Mommy! JEFFFFFFFF!" Christy shouted.

It was on a routine check that Rosalyn came to the bathroom and saw Christy wailing, "JEFFFFFFFF! . . . JEFFFFFFFF!" tears streaming down her cheeks and a red potty ring around her bottom from sitting on it so long. That's where and how they both learned early, as the saying goes, that the job is never done until the paperwork is through.

BEDRIDDEN WITH A PAINFUL KNEE

I was home that day, bedridden with a painful knee injury. Getting up and walking about was pure torture, so I had to depend on the family when I needed something, and more so on Jeff or Christy since I could call them when I needed them. Christy took her responsibilities as my "nurse" very seriously and was usually at my beck and call.

On that particular day, Christy had invited Raya, her friend and the neighbor's little girl, over to play after preschool. The two passed my door going in and out of Christy's room, busy playing.

Eventually, I needed something and called Christy. There was no response. I thought that strange. Perhaps she had not heard me, so I called her name again, louder this time. "CHRISTEEE!" I shouted, "CHRISTEEE!"

Still no response. Raya appeared in the doorway, smiled at me, and left. I was puzzled, and tried again. "CHRISTEEE! CHRISTEEE!" I shouted, louder than before.

Before long Raya reappeared with a piece of paper in her hand. She handed the piece of paper to me. On it, she had scribbled in big, block letters: "CHRISTY IS IN THE BATH-ROOM."

"Oh," I said and thanked her.

DEAF-MUTE

Most deaf people cringe when someone uses the terms "deaf-mute" or "deaf and dumb." In the old days, these words meant a person who could not hear and could not speak. Today, those terms are outdated and considered misnomers, although they still appear occasionally in the press. Not only are these terms inaccurate and archaic, but many people consider them insulting. Deaf people, generally speaking, are not mute. Most have working vocal cords, although they may choose not to use them. They can scream and shout, and if you don't believe me, ask a hearing person who has been a dormitory counselor in a residential school for the deaf!

I am one of those people who wince when I see "deaf-mute" used mistakenly. So it amused my wife to witness my reaction that day she came to visit me in the hospital. I explained to the attending nurse that I was deaf and that it would be very helpful for all concerned if the doctors, nurses, and other hospital personnel were aware of my deafness when they entered my room. At least they would realize that I wasn't ignoring them on purpose! She agreed and offered to put a sign to that effect on my door.

When Rosalyn arrived, she had a smirk on her face. She wanted to know if I had seen the note on the door.

"No," I responded.

"The note reads," my wife signed with a straight face, "'Please note: Patient is deaf and mute.'"

"What!" I exclaimed. "How could she write that after I just *talked* to her?!"

"Oh, you poor deaf-mute," my wife responded mockingly.

I decided to talk with the nurse again. Patiently, I explained that I was not mute. That most deaf people were not mute. I explained how the term originated and how it was so commonly misused. On and on, I went as the nurse listened patiently. When I finished, she offered to "fix it."

The next day when Rosalyn returned for another visit, I detected a suppressed grin on her face. "There is some improvement with the sign," she said.

"Improvement? What do you mean?" I inquired.

"The new note," my wife explained, "reads, 'Note: Patient deaf but not mute.'"

I sighed in desperation, realizing that many of us go through our lives trying to educate others. Considering the progress I was making, I realized I was going to need an awfully long life.

DADDY! GET YOUR ELBOW OFF THE HORN!

Whenever Rosalyn and I went on a long automobile trip when Jeff and Christy were very young, we liked to wake up and get on the road as early as possible. That allowed the children to sleep awhile and gave us the opportunity to cover as much distance as we could, thus shortening the trip somewhat for the kids. It also gave Mom and Dad a few moments of peace and quiet before the kids woke. When we stopped for breakfast, the "How much longer, Mommy?" routine began, and then we started counting the number of restroom stops.

Our trip to St. Louis the summer the kids were six and eight years old was a typical example. We decided to combine business and pleasure on this journey. We were attending the National Association of the Deaf convention in St. Louis, where I was on the program, and then we would drive on down to West Plains to visit my family and the kids' grandparents.

We got up at three a.m., hoping to be on the road by four o'clock. Together we loaded the car in the early morning darkness. When we were ready, I went into the house, carried out Jeff

214

and Christy, and put them in the back of the station wagon, still asleep and snugly wrapped in blankets. Dixie, the family boxer, curled up between them. I checked everything in the house, got two mugs of coffee, locked the house doors, and returned to the car.

As I got into the driver's side and reached over to place coffee in the cupholders in the center of the dashboard, Jeff grabbed my arm and yanked it, causing me to spill some of the coffee. "Hey, quit it!" I yelled, upset, and I wondered what had gotten into that kid. I quickly stepped backed out of the car and looked at Jeff to see what was wrong, but he had laid down and gone back to sleep. I assumed it had been an accident and again started to place the mugs in their holders.

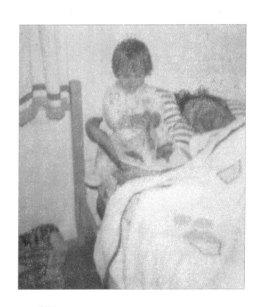

I was supposed to be reading a bedtime story to Christine but instead she read to me as I fell fast asleep, 1978.

As I reached over to place the cups in their holders a second time, Jeff again grabbed my arm and yanked again, causing another coffee spill on the seat. I looked at Jeff again, upset, trying to understand what was wrong.

Jeff quickly signed with a frown and drowsy look: "Daddy! Daddy! Get your elbow off the horn!"

Embarrassed for making so much noise at that ungodly hour, Rosalyn and I hastily departed, wondering what the neighbors thought.

SING ALONG WITH . . . HUH?

Most deaf people who have heard music before will tell you that is what they miss the most. I am one of those people. If I could hear again for a few minutes or for an hour, I would want to hear my children's voices and then listen to music. Long after I became deaf, many of the melodies I once heard linger on. They are cherished memories.

It was early in the morning, and I watched dawn breaking on the horizon as I drove. We were on one of our long trips— Rosalyn was asleep on my side, and the two kids and Dixie were sleeping in the back of the station wagon. I began to feel drowsiness coming on, so to keep awake, I started singing. Once I got going with a song, I began to have visions of myself standing on a stage in the spotlight, my right hand clutching the microphone, my left hand high above my head waving rhythmically in the air, my body bent slightly backward, and my mouth open wide. I imagined myself singing like Perry Como, Bing Crosby, Gene Autry, Frank Sinatra, and others I remembered hearing on the radio as a youth.

I saw Dixie raise her head in the rearview mirror. I ignored her as she perked her ears and tilted her head sideways, trying to decipher the—should I say strange?—sound.

As I continued to sing, the volume swelled up in my expanded chest and carried out over my imaginary audience, which swayed with the rhythm and looked enthralled. I was belting out a tune, and about the time I felt my audience was in a trance, I felt a gentle tapping on my shoulder. I turned my head to look in Jeff's sad, sleepy face. "Please, Daddy, please," he signed, sleepily, "Please be quiet. I want to sleep."

So much for my deaf voice! It had let me down again. I returned my concentration to the long, boring strip of pavement that stretched for miles and miles ahead.

DADDY, WHAT TOOK YOU SOOOOO LONG?!

I was on my hands and knees working in one of the flower beds in the front yard. The cold days of winter had finally passed, and Jeff and Christy and their friends were playing in the backyard, enjoying one of the first warm days of spring. Jeff was then about seven years old and Christy five.

A shadow passed over the area where I was working, which told me someone had approached. I looked up to see Raya, Christy's next-door playmate, standing at my side. She looked at me and smiled shyly. I said a quick hello, not really paying attention, and returned to planting the marigolds.

Some time passed before I looked up again, and to my surprise, Raya was still there watching me. She had more interest in flowers than most kids I knew, I thought to myself. She nodded and said something with her tiny lips, which hardly moved. I didn't understand her and assumed it was just a general comment that little children often made. I smiled, nodded, and went back to planting.

After a while, I felt a light tap on my shoulder and looked up. Raya still stood there, her hands clasped in front of her lap, twisting in a nervous motion. She spoke again, but I still could not understand what she was saying. I have always had difficulty lipreading children, and Raya's lips were impossible. I could not figure out what she wanted. I looked around to see if there was anything unusual. Detecting nothing, I smiled again, nodded, and went back to what I was doing. Raya was about one year younger than Christy, and she was very, very shy. She seldom spoke to me. She had attractive brown eyes and long, black hair, and was a carbon copy of her mother.

More time passed before I straightened up to give my knees and back a break. This time I was startled and alarmed to see Raya still looking at me patiently, prancing back and forth on one foot then on the other. Instinct told me something was amiss. I now knew she was there for a reason.

"Do you want something, Raya?" I asked.

She nodded her head, yes, and pointed in the direction of the back yard and said, "Christy . . ."

I looked at her intently and nodded that I had understood. "Christy, what?" I asked.

"Christy . . . ," she began again, slowly mouthing the words, "Christy stuck . . . stuuuck . . ." all the while nodding for emphasis, " . . . stuuuuck in the tree . . . treeeee . . . treeee. . . ."

I nodded as if she was telling me a story and picked up another marigold . . . then it hit me! I knew Christy was playing in the backyard and she was. . . .

"What?!" I yelped! "Christy! Stuck! Tree! Good God!" My heart did a somersault.

I was on my feet in an instant. I tossed the trowel in one direction and the unplanted marigold in another and bounded through the flower bed I had just planted. I tore around the side of the house toward the backyard faster than I had ever run in my life. My body must have tilted forty-five degrees as I circled the corner of the house. It is a good thing the gate was open, or I would have probably gone right through it.

As I reached the backyard, I could see a shoeless, fat little leg dangling precariously from one of the lower tree branches.

Family, 1997.

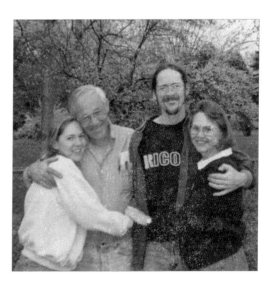

A sneaker lay on the ground. Christy's other leg hung over another branch, which she straddled, and both arms hugged the tree trunk. I grabbed her and eased her to the ground then knelt beside her. I gave her a long, tight hug and thanked the Lord for her safety. I turned around to look for Jeff.

One of our family rules was that the kids had to stay together when they played out of our sight since they could not call us if they needed help. By sticking together, one could always run and get us. But Jeff had forgotten the rule or had assumed that Raya's presence was sufficient. He had hoisted Christy up the tree at her insistence, then wandered off with his chums, forgetting about her. And I hadn't helped either by not paying attention to Raya.

Christy looked up at me, a frightened expression on her face as tears ran down her cheeks. A deep sense of despair and guilt came over me as she signed with her chubby little hands, "Daddy! Daddy!" she hiccupped and scolded, "Daddy, what took you sooooo long?!"

PART FOUR

INTERACTION WITH THE HEARING WORLD AS A DEAF PROFESSIONAL

On His Deafness

My ears are deaf, and yet I seem to hear
Sweet nature's music and the songs of man,
For I have learned from Fancy's artisan
How written words can thrill the inner ear
Just as they move the heart, and so for me
They also seem to ring out loud and free.
In silent study, I have learned to tell
Each secret shade of meaning, and to hear
A magic harmony, at once sincere,
That somehow notes the tinkle of a bell,
The cooing of a dove, the swish of leaves,
The raindrop's pitter-patter on the eaves,
The lover's sigh, the thrumming of guitar—
And if I choose, the rustle of a star!

—Robert F. Panara

Robert F. Panara (1920–2014) was a popular professor at both Gallaudet University and the National Technical Institute for the Deaf (NTID). He was the first deaf professor at NTID. He founded the NTID Drama Club and also was a founding member of the National Theatre of the Deaf. He loved poetry, drama, teaching, and baseball—in about that order. He also was an author. He was born and grew up in New York, where spinal meningitis made him deaf when he was ten years old.

INTRODUCTION

While at Gallaudet, Jack R. Gannon took on a variety of leadership roles with the alumni office and with a succession of university presidents. As the first paid director of alumni relations, he had the task of building connections between the primarily Deaf alumni and a predominantly hearing administration.

Writing volumes, Jack gave presentations to Deaf youth, academic administrators, international visitors, and gatherings of the National Association of the Deaf. His comments often reflected on ways to confront stigma, or what had yet to be called "audism" about the Deaf community. Valuing ASL, Jack often acknowledged Deaf people who had taught him not only language but also how to survive and thrive as a Deaf person. Through decades of service to Gallaudet, he dealt with everyday institutional management while trying to change attitudes.

Jack's love of history and prompting from the National Association of the Deaf led to an intensely complicated research endeavor to write a history of the American Deaf community. In 1981, at the age of forty-five, Jack published a seminal work,

Deaf Heritage: A Narrative History of Deaf America. He quickly became a sought-after presenter, engaged in much international travel to represent the US Deaf community to the wider world.

During these years of rapid change in technology and access, institutions were also changing. Congresses of the World Federation of the Deaf began tipping from primarily hearing-managed events with mostly hearing presenters to events where Deaf people held leadership roles and determined how precious time together would be used at the international meetings. The Deaf President Now movement dramatically shifted the way Gallaudet University would both operate and be seen by the world. The Americans with Disabilities Act signed into law measures of accommodation and access while forging a new spirit of equality. These shifts of power both influenced Jack and were touched by his advocacy.

THE "DEAF NOD"

The "Deaf Nod" is a habit deaf people acquire sooner or later. It is as much a part of our culture as we are. Most of us consider it our escape hatch from insanity.

After many years of frustrating attempts to lipread people and so often encountering unreadable lips, most deaf people develop this immunity system. The Deaf Nod is naturally and quickly learned, and most of the time, is very effective. It has some risks, however. When it fails, it can be utterly embarrassing. It works like this: We nod when someone is talking to us to indicate that we understand when in actuality, we don't. Often, in such situations, to tell the truth, we don't even have the foggiest idea of what the conversation is about. The use of the Deaf Nod is also a gesture of kindness on our part, a consideration of sorts for the poor speaker who would otherwise—if we shook our heads in the negative—keep repeating and repeating and repeating. Admittedly, the Deaf Nod does have one unsurmountable defect that frequently gets us into trouble. If the speaker should question us or throw us a quizzical look, we know we are in deep trouble.

How many times I've used the Deaf Nod I'll never know, but one experience stands out more vividly than all the rest, and, because of what happened, I am now much wiser and much more cautious when I use it. On a trip to Seattle, I was standing on the waterfront of Fisherman's Wharf, enjoying the sights and observing the busy hubbub in the area. Far below, the debris-laden, dark green water of Puget Sound lapped at the wooden pilings. Beer cans, soda-pop bottles, waterlogged boards, paper, and other litter floated on the surface. It was an ugly sight.

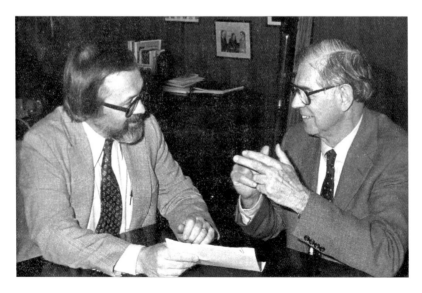

Dr. Edward C. Merrill (right), president of Gallaudet College from 1969 until 1983, and me.

The pier where I stood was U-shaped, providing a berth for the ferries that plied the Sound, transporting cars and people to the islands beyond. Two rows of thick timber pilings bound tightly together with rusting cable ringed the berth. The row facing the water was about five feet lower than the higher row on which I leaned. As I looked down into the dark, murky depths, I wondered to myself what would happen if someone were to fall into the water. There was no ladder, nor any ropes, nor lifesaver rings, nor handholds in sight, and the pilings looked too slippery to climb or grasp. I shuddered at the thought of such a mishap.

I had come to Seattle to participate in the biennial National Association of the Deaf convention. During a break in the proceedings, I had decided to take a stroll down to this popular area. The smell of baked goods penetrated the air where local farmers sold their fruits and vegetables; fishermen marketed their day's catch, and the jewelry and leather makers hawked their wares. It had been an enjoyable and relaxing walk, but now I was tired and leaned on the top of a piling post to rest and enjoy the sights sprawled out before me.

A lively, young, tousled-haired lad wearing a new Seattle T-shirt and sneakers skipped by and stopped not far from where I stood. He must have been ten or eleven years old and was obviously a tourist. He, too, leaned on the pilings and looked below. When he glanced my way, I smiled and nodded in a friendly gesture but said nothing and resumed my relaxed viewing. I was in a quiet mood and wanted to be alone. Out of the corner of my trained eye, however, I realized that the lad was talking to me. I turned to face him and saw his lips moving. He was pointing to something below, and my eyes followed the direction in which he pointed. He had noticed a big dead fish on top of the lower piling. He said something to me that I did not understand, and not wanting to become engaged in a conversation, I gave him the Deaf Nod. I turned my gaze elsewhere. In the distance, I could see a hazy outline of snow-topped Mt. Rainier. After a while, I looked back to where the young boy had stood and was horrified at what I saw. He had climbed over the top piling and was standing on top of the slippery lower pilings. Hugging the top row with his arms, he was slowly inching along toward that dead fish.

"Hey, kid!" I shouted nervously as I ran toward him. I was nearly scared out of my wits. "Come back up here!" I said, grabbing his arms firmly. One slip and he'd be in the foamy brine below, and I had no idea how on earth I would get him out. I helped him climb back over the top. A hurt and puzzled look was on his face.

In my mind's eye, I did a replay of what had happened when he spoke to me moments before. On recall, I saw more clearly the quizzical look on his face, his furrowed forehead, and his raised eyebrows. I had not been paying close attention then, and

I realized now that he had asked me a question. Probably, "Hey, mister, want me to get that fish?" or something to that effect. And, I had given him the Deaf Nod. I had nodded, yes. That answer could have cost him his life.

I promised myself on that very spot that henceforth I would use the Deaf Nod much, much more sparingly. I walked away, shaken.

THE OVERCONFIDENT SALESMAN

A cocky, overconfident salesman walked jauntily into my office unannounced one day, catching me by surprise. Before I could stop him, he launched into a well-rehearsed and lengthy sales pitch. I raised my hand and tried to interrupt him so I could tell him that I was deaf and did not understand what he was saying. It became evident to me that he was used to such interruptions and had developed a technique to ignore them. I wanted to explain to him that without an interpreter, he was actually talking to the wall and wasting his breath and my time, and that it would be better if he wrote me a note, but he gave me no choice. So I just sat there, and politely "listened" to him, and nodded my head as appropriate. He had bypassed my secretary when she momentarily stepped out of the office, and he had no idea to whom he was talking; he only knew I was the director of the university's alumni and public relations program. Had he given me the opportunity I would have tracked down my secretary, who signed very well, and at least heard him out.

When I tried to say something, he quickly held up his finger, signaling me to wait. I tried again to interrupt, but he only talked faster. Suddenly, the amusement of the situation struck me, so I leaned back in my chair and just sat there, watching his performance, studying his expressions and body language, and not understanding one word he was saying. He mistakenly mistook my behavior as a sign of interest, and encouraged, he enthusiastically continued his lengthy spiel while I sat there bemused. Finally, after a long, wordy presentation, he reached the query part of his talk. The expression on his face, his furrowed forehead, and raised eyebrows told me he had moved into the question phase. He was becoming puzzled as to why he wasn't getting an answer. I was quite sure from past dealings with salespeople that he wanted to know if we were interested in trying his product, what our specific needs were, and how he could be of service to us. Naturally, I didn't answer.

At long last, he stopped talking. His animated body language came to a halt, and a puzzled, quizzical look slowly crept across his face. I could see he was beginning to sense something was wrong.

"I am sorry," I said, "but I am deaf."

"You're what . . . ?" I lipread as he stammered.

"Deaf . . . deaf!" I repeated slowly.

"Deaf? Deaf?!" He imitated. "You're deaf!" he said, pointing his finger at me. "But . . . but . . . I talked to you on the telephone." Indeed, he had. With the assistance of my secretary, who had interpreted his conversation, I had verbally responded to his call. Many deaf people with understandable speech do that.

"You're deaf?" he asked again. When I nodded my head in the affirmative, his chin dropped, and a look of disbelief crept across his face. His body sagged, and his cocky, overconfident attitude seemed to drain out of his body through the soles of his shoes as if he had just sprung a leak. Deflated, he slumped into the nearest chair.

I felt I had a casualty on my hands and was trying to determine what to do next when my secretary walked into the room. She saw the uninvited visitor, gave him a dirty look, glanced my way, and quickly detected the amused grin on my face.

With her interpreting, I extended him the courtesy of explaining the purpose of his visit and repeating his sales pitch. I couldn't help noting how much briefer it was. He quickly left the office, much wiser, I hope, from the experience.

MAC AND HIS METAL BEDPAN

My friend, Mac, had been admitted to the hospital for a very serious illness. On the day I visited him, I noticed his temper was intact and in good health. He was still fuming about an incident that had happened the day before. He had experienced pain and needed assistance, so he called the nurse. You know how the hospital system works. You reach over and press the button on a little device pinned to the side of the bed. Pressing the button signals the nurses' station down the hall, and a light flashes above the patient's bed number to get the nurse's attention.

Mac reached over and pushed his button and waited.

When Mac's bed light went on down at the nurses' station, the attending nurse quickly flipped on the intercom switch to Mac's room and said, "Hello, sir. May I help you?" She was the new shift nurse, and either did not remember or did not know Mac was deaf.

Mac lay back in his bed and waited and waited. Of course, he didn't hear her voice on the intercom over his bed. Although we deaf people have come a long, long way, lipreading an intercom speaker hasn't yet been one of our achievements.

Back at the nurses' station, the nurse waited for a response. Not receiving one, she assumed that her patient had either fallen asleep or no longer needed her assistance, and she flicked off the signal light. She turned her attention back to what she had been doing.

Mac impatiently watched the minute hand on the wall clock and waited. After a while, he pushed the nurse's button again, and the same thing happened.

"Hello, sir, can I help you?" the nurse asked, speaking into the intercom. "Hello, sir, is there something I can get you?" Receiving no response, she shrugged her shoulders and resumed her work.

Down the hall, Mac was becoming increasingly upset. His adrenaline began to surge with each tick of the minute hand on the wall clock. He jammed the button again and again . . . and waited . . . and waited. . . .

At that point, however, the attending nurse had left the nurses' station to respond to another patient's call. Mac had no way of knowing that. The longer he waited, the angrier he became. Finally, he erupted in a rage. He grabbed the metal bedpan beside his bed and flung it across the room. It clattered across the tile floor, crashed into the wall, bounced off, and screeched out into the hallway. *Crash! Bang! Clatter!* Five nurses came running in.

Sorry, sometimes it is necessary for us deaf people to throw our bedpans to get some attention in this hearing world.

I'LL ALWAYS REMEMBER MONIQUE

I'll always remember Monique, the little girl in the kindergarten class at St. Mary's School for the Deaf in Buffalo, New York. I was at the school for a Gallaudet alumni speaking engagement when I met her.

As I entered the classroom that morning, I saw four little girls seated around a low, round, worktable with their teacher and a teacher's aide. The other students in the class, I was told, were out sick. I walked over to the group with my host and sat down in one of the little chairs and joined them. The chair was so low that my knees folded upward almost as high as my chest.

The teacher introduced me to the children and told them that I was from Gallaudet University in Washington, DC, "where the president of the United States lives." She explained that I had flown to Buffalo on an airplane and showed them a picture of a big jet. The little girls nodded in unison, expressions of interest on their faces. They seemed impressed.

"Good morning," I signed as I spoke and looked at each little girl. I thought I would take the initiative and get a dialogue going. Pointing to the first little girl on my left, I asked: "What is your name?" That was always an easy and comfortable way to start a conversation with young deaf children. It was a clincher, and one couldn't go wrong with that approach . . . or so I thought.

Instead of a cheerful and polite response and a "My name is . . ." answer as I expected, the first little girl decided to play a game with me and have some fun. A mischievous look crept over her face. She smiled, then began rocking her head sideways, jutted out her chin defiantly, and signed: SECRET! NOT TELLING YOU!

I was dumbfounded. She caught me off guard. This had never happened to me before! My eyebrows shot up, and I couldn't hide the surprised look on my face. How do you argue with a five-year-old who doesn't want to tell you her name?

I tried to keep my cool. Teasing her, I asked: "Oh, did your Mommy and Daddy forget to give you a name?" But she didn't fall for this.

NO! she signed, stomping her foot on the floor for added emphasis. SECRET! she signed, rocking her head again. The "I'm-not-telling-you" look convinced me she meant business.

There was nothing I could do with Little Miss Stubborn, so with a visual facial sigh, I moved on to the next tot. "Tell me, what is your name?" I signed as I pointed to the next little girl in the circle. Much to my chagrin, she, too, decided to play the game with me and follow Little Miss Stubborn's lead, and I encountered another Little Miss No Name. Once again, I saw another mischievous look, another defiant rocking of the head.

I looked lamely at the teacher and the teacher's aide on my right, and we exchanged weak smiles. As the father of two small fry at that time, I knew what they knew, and they knew what I knew. I was in a hopeless situation. If those youngsters with minds of their own didn't want to tell me anything, there wasn't much I could do.

I took a swallow and turned back to the group. What a way to begin a conversation. What a way to begin the day! A queasy feeling crept into my stomach. In a feeble attempt to save face, I teasingly scolded the two little girls: "When you go home this Friday, I want you to tell your mother and father to give you a name because all little boys and girls I know have names. You understand?" Two little heads bobbed sideways, in defiance. I had just lost another round.

Dread filled my stomach as I moved on to the next child, wondering what I would do if I drew another blank. She was a thin little girl with beautiful, sandy-blonde hair and pretty blue eyes. I later learned that shortly after her birth, her deafness was misdiagnosed as "mental retardation" because she did not respond to the spoken word—not an uncommon occurrence at the time with young deaf children. She was mistakenly placed in a program for children with cognitive developmental issues. She would probably still be in an institution if not for an alert teacher who had become suspicious of her behavior and discovered that she simply was deaf. She was transferred to St. Mary's School in Buffalo, NY, and her teachers were amazed and pleased with her fast adjustment and good progress.

Reluctantly, I pointed to her and asked, "Do you have a name?" When I spoke to her, her face lit up and changed into a beautiful, happy smile, and she nodded her head shyly. Very slowly, she signed and fingerspelled: "My name is M-O-N-I-Q-U-E. I am six years old." She did something that not only saved my day but made me feel warm and welcome and earned her a permanent place in my heart of happy memories. She got up from her small chair, walked around the table, and stopped beside me. Next, she put her small arms around my neck, hugged me, and planted a kiss on my cheek.

DOWN THE STAIRS WITH YERKER

Yerker, a tall, slim, bearded Swede, was one of my best friends. He and his younger brother were born deaf, and they grew up and were educated in Sweden. The cause of their deafness was unknown. Neither had usable speech. Yerker's brother, Savante, became a successful businessman, and Yerker was a professor at Gallaudet University.

Both of Yerker's parents were teachers. His father was superintendent of the local school system, an author, and the founder of a museum in Vallent, a small village north of Stockholm, where they lived. Yerker told me that his father was so well-known in that village that Yerker was required to doff his hat to every adult he passed. He did that so often that within a year, he had a hole in his hat.

Following graduation from school, Yerker became a dental technician and toured Europe on a bicycle. He became very active in deaf organizations in Stockholm. Later he became involved with the World Federation of the Deaf and eventually was elected president of that organization. He knew Swedish and English and was a fluent user of Swedish Sign Language and ASL. Many people considered him to be an expert at Gestuno, a collection of international signs. He also read Danish and Norwegian and could understand French, German, and Dutch. He was the third person from Sweden to graduate from Gallaudet University, where he founded and served as chair of Gallaudet's Department of Deaf Studies before he retired.

We met at Gallaudet as undergraduates, and fate brought us both back to the campus to work.

Yerker and his wife Nancy purchased an old rowhouse in southeast Washington, DC, not far from the Gallaudet campus, and they spent much of their free time remodeling it. I offered to help whenever I was needed. One day Yerker took me up on that offer and asked if I would help him remove some very heavy, old, cast iron radiators from the house. "Sure!" I said, glad to give a friend a hand. The radiators were on the second floor. Yerker wanted to take them downstairs and place them on the front porch, where a scrap dealer had agreed to pick them up.

We lugged the heaviest radiator to the top of the stairway landing with little difficulty. Yerker, taller than me, took the lead and positioned himself in front of the radiator, and I followed it at the other end. We started down the long flight of steps, each of us gripping the heavy radiator with both hands. No sooner had we begun than my feet slipped out from under me and shot up into the air. I landed on a step on the seat of my pants, still holding tightly to the radiator. I couldn't let go of it or it would fall on Yerker, sending him hurtling down the stairs, and seriously injuring him.

I went down each step, dragged by the weight, struggling to straighten up and get my footing back under me, but to no avail. Yerker, in front of the radiator, had his head down, his shoulder bent against the front of the radiator to steady it and hold back the weight. He couldn't look up and see what was going on above him. His attention was focused on each step below him as he carefully guided the radiator down. He was taking extra care so that the radiator would not scratch the wall or touch the banister railings.

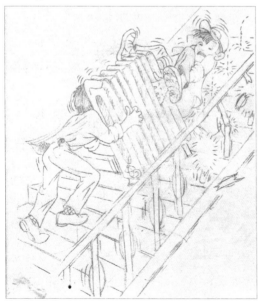

Helping Yerker carry the radiator down the steps, as illustrated by Ruth Peterson.

Thump! Thump! Thump! the radiator and I went down the steps.

There was no point for me to yell because he couldn't hear me, and I couldn't wave and catch his attention because I couldn't let go of the radiator. Neither could I stomp my feet because both feet were flailing in the air.

Thump! Thump! Thump! I bounced down each step on my bottom.

About midway down the stairs, much to my horror, one of the radiator legs started to jut out sideways and catch the stairway rail supports. Instead of snagging and stopping us, as I had hoped, the weight of the radiator started snapping or knocking out the supports. One by one, the supports went flying, either breaking or being knocked from their mounting.

Snap! Thump! Snap! down the stairs Yerker, the radiator, and I went. I could only look on dejectedly as I bounced down those steps furiously holding onto the radiator. Meanwhile, Yerker cautiously guided his end of the radiator smoothly down, unaware of the mayhem taking place above him.

We finally reached the first-floor landing.

Yerker straightened up, smiling, and looking very pleased that the hard part of the task was over and that we had made it to the bottom without incident. Then he looked up and stared aghast at the damage the radiator legs had wrought. He stood with his mouth open, shock on his face, and began shaking his head slowly. I sat on the bottom step on my beaten buttocks, glumly looking from Yerker to the mess I had helped cause.

"What happened?!" Yerker signed with one hand.

"I slipped," I told him.

"Why didn't you tell me?" he asked.

"How?" I responded.

He nodded his head slowly. He understood.

"MOM'S NOW A LITTLE DEAF"

Mel Carter Jr. told me this story. It took place when he was teaching at the North Carolina School for the Deaf in Greensboro.

One of the boys in his class of fourth-graders, unlike most of his students, didn't look forward to going home on weekends. Mel thought that unusual, and a bit strange, and after a little prodding discovered the reason. It turned out that the boy was frustrated by the lack of communication within his family.

BORED! signed the little fellow in exasperation. HOME BOR-ING! he repeated for emphasis.

Mel was touched by the child's plight, which he knew was not uncommon. In fact, he felt it was often too prevalent. He knew the family lived in a rural area and suspected that the boy had few playmates close by. But lack of family communication made the situation much worse.

Mel decided to have a private talk with the boy's mother when she returned to school the following weekend to take her son home. Mel noticed the mother stiffen when he brought up the subject, and she displayed resistance to the idea of learning sign language for various reasons. She was concerned about the impact sign language would have on her son's speech development and felt that speech and lipreading were better or sufficient. She felt that sign language was just a collection of wild gestures and that she could not learn it. Mel asked her if the family's speech and the boy's lipreading skills were sufficient to carry on a comfortable conversation or whether they exchanged just a few brief words here and there. The mother nodded her head slightly but did not respond. Mel then pointed out that ASL was a legitimate language in its own right. He gave her a publisher's catalog and identified the growing collection of sign language books that were coming out. He reminded the mother that her son was a member of the family too, and her son had a right and a need to have access to family conversations, and to be able to communicate freely within his own home. The mother nodded her head, thanked Mel for the meeting, said she would think about it, and left without making any other commitments.

Months passed. Christmas came and went, and the students returned to school in January.

Mel was to learn later that the mother had agonized over the matter for a long time. She talked to other mothers who signed to their children. She knew there was a deaf employee in the factory where she worked whom she had never met. One day she went over and introduced herself and told the deaf woman that she had a deaf son. They began talking with each other. The young deaf coworker told the mother about her own experience growing up in a family where communicating was so difficult and frustrating, and volunteered to teach her sign language. With some hesitancy, the mother agreed and was surprised at how easy it was to learn. After a few lessons, the mother decided to learn sign language as a Christmas surprise for her son. The mother and the deaf coworker began getting together during their lunch hours, and to her surprise she could understand many of the words the deaf woman spoke as she signed.

On Christmas morning, as the family gathered around the Christmas tree, the mother started signing to her son, MERRY CHRISTMAS! MERRY CHRISTMAS! The little boy's eyes grew big and his mouth opened in surprise.

On the first day back at school, the young fellow burst into Mel's classroom beaming. He couldn't wait to tell Mel the good news.

KNOW WHAT? he signed to Mel. Mel shook his head. The boy said, MY MOM NOW A LITTLE DEAF.

TWO LADIES OF THE NIGHT

I had come down to Tampa Bay, Florida, for a weekend with Gary Olsen, executive director of the National Association of the Deaf, and Jim Cox, director of the continuing education program at Gallaudet University. We were the trainers of a regional leadership training program for deaf adults cosponsored by Gallaudet University and the National Association of the Deaf.

It was late—a bit past midnight—and I had just finished my last presentation. I was tired and anxious to get to my room on the fifth floor of the hotel. I walked to the elevators, set my briefcase down, and shifted all my presentation materials to one arm. Out of the corner of my eye, I saw two women in tight-fitting, colorful leotards, five-inch high heels, and heavy makeup, and I guessed they were ladies of the night. It was my first encounter with some professionals in the world's oldest trade. I quickly pushed the UP elevator button with my free hand and waited.

Unfortunately for me, it was one of those instances when the elevator decided to take its good time in arriving. As I stood there waiting, I began to feel uncomfortable as I sensed that the ladies smoking in the corner were looking directly at me. I felt silly just standing there, staring at the elevator door, so I tried to appear calm and collected as I nonchalantly gazed about the lobby area. I was right. I could see they were staring at me, and my deaf instinct told me they had also spoken to me. I ignored them and pushed the elevator button again.

No one else was in the area, and I began to feel increasingly uneasy, but I tried hard not to appear so. With no elevator in sight, I casually looked their way, smiled, nodded my head in greeting, and pushed the danged elevator UP button . . . again.

The next time I looked their way, I could see their mouths moving. The expressions on their faces—furrowed foreheads and arched eyebrows—confirmed that they had been talking to me, most likely asking questions. Locked in their gaze, I had the choice of either looking away coldly and snubbing them or responding. Contrary to what my deafness sometimes makes me appear to be doing, I don't intentionally snub people, so instead, I gave them my standard routine: I pointed a forefinger to one ear, shook my head, and said, "I am deaf."

To my surprise, the one with the dyed blond hair nodded her head knowingly and using a mixture of crude homemade signs and the two-handed British manual alphabet responded: "We know. Where are you from?"

I glanced apprehensively back to the slow elevator, looking—
and hoping—for an excuse to interrupt the conversation before
it began, but found none. My elevator had apparently gotten lost.
I felt the only thing to do was to suppress my anxiety and go talk
with them. I walked over to the corner, put my load of materials
down, and answered her question. Both nodded their heads in
acknowledgment, giving me the impression they already knew
about the meeting. I suspected they had been informed about
this group of deaf out-of-towners meeting at the hotel and
had wandered over to check out the business since one of them
"spoke"—up to a point—our language a little bit.

It was natural for me to ask the one who signed where she
had learned her sign language. She told me she had learned
some signs from a deaf childhood friend, some at church, and
had invented the rest, which was quite obvious to me. While
not accurate, her mouthing the words and using her crude signs
simultaneously were sufficient to carry on a simple conversation.

Suddenly, they both pointed in the direction of the elevators.
The door of my long-awaited elevator finally opened, giving me
the opportunity to excuse myself and avoid getting into a deeper
conversation. I grabbed my stack of materials and explained I
had to go.

As I headed for the elevator, the blonde signed to me: "Good
night. I will pray for you."

I nodded my head in acknowledgment, then puzzled, asked, "Why?"

"So you can hear someday," she responded.

"Thanks," I said expressing my appreciation for her concern, "but I am very happy the way I am."

As the elevator ascended to the fifth floor, I thought about her offer to pray for me and wondered to myself who needed the prayer more.

THROUGH THE MAZE WITH THE POTTY PATROL

Following a regional workshop on deafness in Tulsa, Oklahoma, a group of us deaf and hearing educators, rehabilitation counselors, parents of deaf children, deaf consumers, and interpreters decided to go out for dinner. The restaurant a local had recommended appeared most intriguing. The interior of the restaurant was dark and very uniquely designed. Instead of one large room, it had been divided into a maze of many small eating areas, with each area separated from the other by short partitions, which were decorated with posters, pictures, and antiques. Large plants hung overhead.

The waiters were outrageously dressed. They wore everything and anything imaginable. They were dressed like hobos, clowns, football players, molls, dolls, and gangsters and what have you.

On our arrival, the restaurant host led us through the maze of eating areas to our table, which appeared to be somewhere in a corner in the back. After everyone had ordered, Bob, one of the deaf participants, had to go to the restroom. But where were they?! He stood up at the table and looked around the darkened maze of enclosed tables and partitions packed with people, and correctly surmised that he couldn't go more than twenty feet before he would be lost. So he did the smart thing—he asked his waiter for directions to the men's room.

On hearing the word "restroom," our waiter instantly changed his behavior. He straightened up, stiffened, and adopted first a funny facial expression, then a very dignified look. His attempt at appearing dignified clashed with his ridiculous apparel. He raised his index finger and beseeched Bob for a little patience as he signaled for another employee. When the second employee arrived, our waiter explained solemnly to Bob (with a colleague interpreting) that this second employee had the most important responsibility in the whole restaurant. Everyone at our table eyed the new person, puzzled. He wore tuxedo tails over a torn T-shirt. A black bow tie was strapped around his neck. His faded jeans were a couple of inches short of his ankles, and he wore black tennis shoes without socks, of course. His responsibility? Leading patrons to the appropriate restroom!

Bob looked at the others at our table and raised his eyebrows, wondering what they were up to. But, he had to go, and when you have to go, you have to go. He stood up, and Mr. Restroom Finder grabbed one of Bob's hands and placed it on his shoulder. A look of embarrassment crept over Bob's face, and it was obvious that he felt silly, but he had a more pressing need—to find the restroom—and decided to go along with the act, whatever it was. Next, Mr. Restroom Finder raised his leg knee-high, started marching, and commanded Bob to follow suit. Then, the leader raised both arms in the air and started shouting loud enough for all the patrons to hear—except the deaf ones, of course. With his hands on the leader's shoulder, Bob could feel the vibrations and knew he was talking, but had no idea what he was saying. Bob looked at the customers and was puzzled when he realized they were bellowing with laugher. He thought that perhaps it was the sight of this silly marching spectacle that was funny, and deciding to be a good sport, smiled back. Off the two went, marching through the maze of tables in an exaggerated search for the restroom. Everyone laughed except us deaf people who looked on amused at the sight, but not really knowing what was fully going on.

When Bob eventually found his way back to our table, a hearing colleague explained what had happened. As the two of them marched to the restroom, with Bob's hands on his shoulders, the leader sang loudly:

"Here comes the potty patrol, the potty patrol!
Hey, make way! Hey, make way! Hey, make way!
For the potty patrol . . . the potty patrol!
Hey! Here comes the potty patrol, the potty patrol!"

The urge to go to the restroom among the rest of us suddenly disappeared!

"ALWAYS ON FRIDAY"

I had returned to NSD for a speaking engagement. I was taking a break from my visit with the students and teachers and was sitting in the teachers' lounge one Friday afternoon, recalling the years when Rosalyn and I were teachers there and the many young boys and girls we had worked with and gotten to know personally. I also thought about the teachers we had taught with, and the wonderful times we had shared. In the midst of my reverie, big, burly Neal walked in.

Neal was one of my former students and had been a great football player. At five-eleven and close to three hundred pounds, he had been one of the huskiest players I had ever had on any of my teams. He played right guard on our eight-man football team and was almost big enough to fill two slots in the line. He was very strong. I wasn't exactly a weakling myself. I had played college football, but when Neal came up behind me on the football field during practice, as he liked to do, caught me by surprise in a double-arm grip and lifted me off the ground, I was helpless. Neal would then turn around slowly in front of all the players with me locked in his grip, and smile broadly as the players guffawed in delight to see their coach's feet dangling off the ground like a wet towel.

Neal was a lovable guy. He was one of our "low-achievers." What he lacked in academics, he made up in happiness, good cheer, and hard work. There was always that ear-to-ear grin on his big, round face. It seemed he couldn't get mad at anyone even if he tried.

When Neal was an infant, his family was involved in a tragic automobile accident that killed his younger sister. Neal was thrown from the car, and his head hit the pavement, I was told, causing brain damage and possibly his deafness and learning disabilities. He was deeply attached to his family, and that may have accounted for the only problem I had ever had with him as a coach.

Most of our football games were played on Fridays, and many of the boys would go home afterward. Once in a while, we had a game on a Saturday, and that required a change in plans. It created transportation and other problems if the boys did not stay overnight at the school. While the other players enjoyed staying on campus during the weekend, usually filled with teen activities, Neal didn't relish the idea. He was different. He insisted on going home every Friday.

One particular week we had an important game coming up with a school a great distance from ours. It was an away game, and because of a scheduling conflict, it had been rescheduled for a Saturday. I had asked the players to remain overnight at the school so we could get an early Saturday morning start.

Following the final workout that week, we held our regular pregame team briefing. That was when Neal dropped his bomb. At the end of the meeting, I asked the players if they had any questions. Neal slowly raised his hand to get my attention and signed, "I can't play Saturday."

"What?!" I exclaimed, startled. This was no time to learn that my starting guard was going to be absent the day after tomorrow. Concerned that a family emergency had come up or some other dreadful event had occurred, I nervously asked, "Why? What happened, Neal?"

"I go home on Fridays," he informed me matter-of-factly.

"I know," I responded. I didn't see that as a problem, "But we have an important game Saturday. I want you to play. You can go home after the game. Okay?"

"I know," Neal signed, "but I go home on Fridays."

I tried not to let Neal see how upset I was becoming. "We need you, Neal. You are part of the team. We can't win without you!"

"I know," Neal responded calmly, nodding his head in agreement. Then, he lowered his eyes to the floor, as if he were ashamed to look at me, "but I *always* go home on Friday."

Oh Lord, I thought. What would I do? I was frantic. We had practiced all week with him in that position. We did not have a good substitute to replace him. I reasoned and pleaded with him. I got his teammates to talk with him and to coax him to change his mind, all to no avail. Desperate, I ran to the principal's office and explained my plight. The principal was sympathetic and shared my concern. He offered to call Neal's parents, who lived in a distant city, to see if something could be worked out. They offered to make the long trip to the school, pick Neal up as usual on Friday afternoon, take him home, then drive him to the game early Saturday morning and meet us there. I was relieved. Things worked out after all, and, yes, we won that game.

Here in the lounge, I was reliving that incident when—speak of the devil—Neal walked in. Big, broad, smiling, happy Neal. We greeted each other with bear hugs and, like old times, Neal's arms locked around me, and he lifted me off the floor. When he finally put me down, I took a good look at him. He was now a grown man and much heavier than before. I invited him to join me for a soda and a chat. I asked him what he was doing, and he told me proudly that he was now the school custodian. Very seriously, and in great detail, he explained to me all his job responsibilities and how he performed each task. When he was finally through, I knew the school building was in good hands. He also told me that he was "still a bachelor" and that he had his own apartment near the school. I asked about his parents, and he told me how they were doing. He also explained that he had entered into a partnership with a boyhood friend in his hometown and that together they raised and sold horses on the side.

"We have ninety-nine horses now," he signed proudly, displaying his ear-to-ear grin.

"Wow!" I signed, shaking my right hand, impressed. "What do you do with so many horses?"

"We breed them, raise them, and sell them," he signed, still beaming with pride.

I was pleased to know that despite all the difficulties Neal had encountered as a youth, he was now a proud, self-supporting citizen of Nebraska and leading an independent, successful life. He was a credit to the school and to his teachers, whose patience and understanding had brought out the best in him. Now he was working, paying his share of taxes, and repaying the state that had supported this school and made his education possible. In his own way, he was another NSD success story.

My break time had expired, and I had to get back on schedule. I got up to leave and bade Neal farewell. As I was going, I had an afterthought, and I turned and asked him: "You coming to my talk tonight, Neal?" I knew many members of the Deaf community would be there, and I thought I might remind him. But, to my surprise, he shook his head quickly and asked, "You forget?"

I was disappointed and surprised but decided not to say anything. He saw the look on my face and responded with a perplexed expression as if to say, "Don't you remember?" He then signed, "I *always* go home on Fridays."

CARLOS KEEPS ME TIMED

Many deaf kids use the sign for "finish" at the end of each sentence or thought sequence to let the receiver know they've made their point and are ready to move on. This way, if the recipient hasn't understood the message, the signer can repeat it before proceeding. Many young deaf kids will, therefore, sign something, stop, sign FINISH, raise their eyebrows in a questioning expression, and look at whomever they're talking to in order to be sure they are being followed before they proceed.

But FINISH, or for added emphasis FINISH! FINISH!—waving the spread fingers of the hand in a snapping motion—has another meaning. It means, "Enough! Enough! Stop! Stop! Finish! Finish!" Or, sometimes, it comes across as a warning, like when a supervisor tells students to stop whatever they are doing.

I was invited to the Mill Neck Manor Lutheran School for the Deaf to talk about *Deaf Heritage* and my latest book, *The Week the World Heard Gallaudet.* My hostess, Maria Lemperis, who was the Total Communication coordinator, shared with me a copy of "Anthology 1990" that the children had written. The collection included prose and poetry, and those children who did not have sufficient language to make a contribution had submitted artwork. It was a collection that represented the entire school.

My interaction with the young children before the presentation began quickly told me that some of them had no language at all. But their communication was expressed on their faces, in their eyes, in the attention they gave me or didn't give me, and in their smiles. Some of the children came from other countries and didn't know English. Others were a smart bunch who would ask the most questions and prod me for more details to savor my stories and make them last as long as possible.

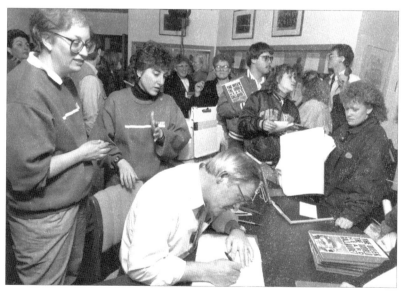

Autographing my book The Week the World Heard Gallaudet, *1989.*

One of my new friends, Carlos, sat there on the floor in front of me with his legs crossed and his hands resting on his ankles. He wore a white paper Earth Day cap. Carlos and his family, I learned afterward, had moved to New York from El Salvador less than a year before, and he had only been enrolled in the school since the previous summer. He was eight years old and learning three languages almost simultaneously! His home language was spoken Spanish, he was learning English in school, and he was picking up ASL. While his expressive signing skills were developing well, it was clear to me that his receptive skills were not sufficient for him to fully understand me. So, while I gave my presentation, Carlos and I had a private conversation.

Before I began, Carlos signed to me, TALK, TALK, FINISH, LUNCH. LUNCH FINISH, PLAY. PLAY FINISH, SCHOOL, SCHOOL FINISH, HOME. He signed with a broad smile on his face. After he told me that, he raised his eyebrows and nodded his head with a question mark on his face. "You get the idea?" his expression was asking me. Then it dawned on me. Carlos was trying to familiarize me with the school routine so I wouldn't foul up. He wanted to be sure I did not talk past lunchtime. I nodded my head to him that I understood . . . and nobody else knew what was going on!

While I spoke, it saddened me to see the familiar blank stare of incomprehension on many of the children's faces, but bless them—they extended to me the courtesy of their attention even though they did not understand most of what I was saying. One little boy waved his hand to get my attention. He had multiple disabilities, and he had almost no language. The vocabulary he had was inconsistent. HOME, CAR, MOTHER, FATHER, he told me. He was able to pick out those four words or signs I had used and wanted me to know that at his house, his parents also had a car. I smiled in acknowledgment and signed, "Really! That's great!"

Another little girl raised her hand and asked why the patrolman hadn't given my friend a ticket. "Why do you think he didn't give him a ticket?" I repeated. Different children had different answers. Then the girl who had asked the question first gave the answer. "Forgot?" she queried. "Yes," I responded. "I think he forgot, too."

When I looked his way again, Carlos returned my look with a frown on his face "You're long!" he told me disapprovingly. Then he signed, "I'm hungry!" with a forlorn look on his face.

Following my presentation to the adults that evening, I was approached by an elderly woman who turned out to be the mother of a deaf friend of mine. She was concerned about the speech development of her two granddaughters. "It's a hearing world out there," she told me. I knew the girls. They were in the morning group I had spoken to, and they had asked very good questions. I had visited their home when they were younger and was amazed at how sharp and smart they were, but grandma seemed only concerned about their speech development. I asked if she realized that her granddaughters were probably the smartest kids in the school! She nodded her head and said, "but it's a hearing world out there." I couldn't resist. "Does the world out there belong only to hearing people?" I asked.

To my surprise, she thanked me for what I was doing for deaf Americans, and then she left. I was upset and saddened. She was the mother of a deaf friend. She could follow my presentation because I had used my speech as I signed, yet I had to use an interpreter to understand her. It didn't matter that

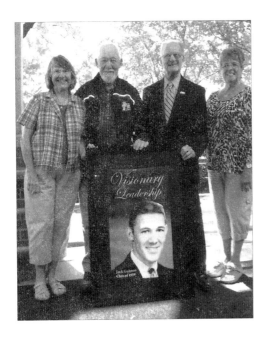

Dr. Alan Hurwitz, former president of Gallaudet, presented me with a framed banner during Gallaudet's sesquicentennial, with Rosalyn (far left) and Dr. Hurwitz's wife, Vicki (far right).

her grandchildren were smart, doing well in school, excelling in sports, and receiving job training. As far as she was concerned, if the children didn't have speech, they were doomed. Sadly, she was not alone. All my deaf friends and I knew the advantage of good speech, but it often appeared to us that those hearing people who pushed only speech were the most insensitive and damaging when it came to communicating with deaf people. Many would not bother to include us in a conversation. They were often very patronizing, and few would share tidbits of information of what was being said in a group conversation. We were not full participants in family or social gatherings; we were left on the fringes at the mercy of our hearing "friends." With sign language, we were equals and fuller participants regardless of whether the other person was deaf or hearing.

ABOUT THE AUTHOR

Through this personal collection of stories, readers have a window into the ways Jack R. Gannon's life has been shaped by the places and people encountered along his journey: West Plains, Missouri; Richmond, California; Fulton, Missouri; Omaha, Nebraska; and Washington, DC. His extensive national and international travels brought him into contact with diverse peoples and provided fertile ground for learning different ways of living. An intense observer of human nature, Jack shares in this book revealing interactions with strangers and friends, as well as beloved family stories on the joys, challenges, and humor in raising children—in this case, hearing children.

As a teacher, coach, and university administrator, Jack built an impressive record of service, but it is his contributions to Deaf history that are most often noted. A curator, an author, and a historian, Jack has long been a cultural bridge between Deaf and hearing people. His numerous books serve as resources for intercultural sharing and have earned him honors including the National Association of the Deaf Distinguished Service Award and the Edward Allen Fay Award from the Conference of Educational Administrators of Schools and Programs for the Deaf. Jack received an honorary doctorate from Gallaudet University where he was also inducted into the university hall of fame and named a Sesquicentennial Visionary Leader. The World Federation of the Deaf bestowed the International Solidarity Merit Award, First Class, to Jack and Rosalyn Gannon for immeasurable contributions to global Deaf communities.

Connecting with people comes naturally to Jack, and from a few of these stories, you will see that he is not shy about com-

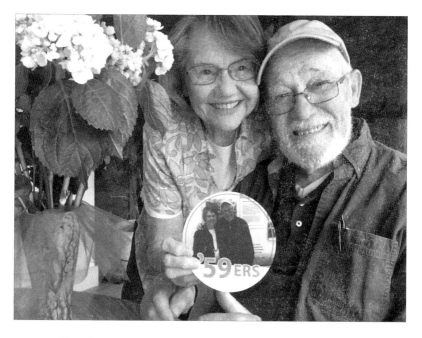

Rosalyn and I celebrating our sixtieth wedding anniversary.

municating with nonsigners. He always makes the effort to engage with everyone and has shared a scribbled conversation with countless hearing people. Rarely did they know the cultural gift he has been to the Deaf community.

Jack and Rosalyn Gannon, married for more than sixty years, live in an eighteenth-century farmhouse in New Market, Maryland.

—Jean L. Bergey

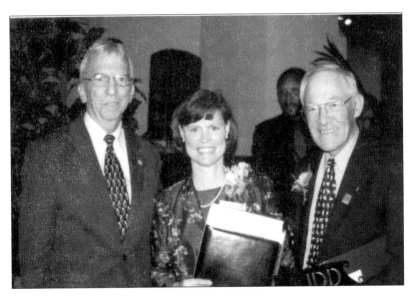

Former Gallaudet President I. King Jordan and Jean L. Bergey with me at the 2002 opening of the History through Deaf Eyes *exhibit at the Smithsonian Institution.*

Other books by Jack R. Gannon:

The Week the World Heard Gallaudet
Deaf Heritage: A Narrative History of Deaf America
Through Deaf Eyes: A Photographic History of an
    American Community (coauthored with Douglas C. Baynton and Jean L. Bergey)
World Federation of the Deaf: A History